License Practical Nurse Practice Exam Reviewer

M.A Gorre

Disclaimer

Disclaimer

This Practice Exam Reviewer for the CLPN Exam ("Reviewer") is intended for study and preparation purposes only and is in no way affiliated with, or endorsed by, the official Certified Licensed Practical Nurse (CLPN) examination body or any other official body. The creator of this Reviewer has made every effort to ensure the accuracy and completeness of the information provided. However, neither the creator nor the distributor makes any warranties, expressed or implied, regarding the accuracy, adequacy, completeness, legality, reliability, or usefulness of any information, and they expressly disclaim liability for errors and omissions in the contents of this Reviewer.

No Guarantee of Passing

The usage of this Reviewer does not guarantee the passing of any exams, and it is the user's responsibility to use multiple study aids and refer to the official examination guidelines and materials to prepare adequately for the CLPN Exam. It is also the responsibility of the user to comply with all applicable laws, regulations, and policies regarding exam preparation and participation.

Intellectual Property Rights

This Reviewer may contain questions that are similar to those that may appear in the official exam, but they are original creations of the author and any resemblance to actual past exam questions is coincidental. Unauthorized copying, distribution, or transmission of this Reviewer, or any portion thereof, is strictly prohibited.

Indemnification

Users agree to indemnify and hold harmless the creator and distributor of this Reviewer from and against any and all claims, demands, liabilities, costs or expenses, including reasonable attorney's fees, arising out of or in connection with the use of this Reviewer or breach of this Disclaimer.

Usage of Reviewer

This Reviewer is created for educational purposes, and users may purchase it for personal use only. Any redistribution, reselling, or public dissemination of the Reviewer or any of its contents without the express written consent of the author is strictly prohibited. Users are advised to use the information contained in this Reviewer at their own discretion and risk.

By purchasing or using this Reviewer, you acknowledge and agree to this disclaimer and assume full responsibility for the use of this product.

Commercial Rights

The author retains all commercial rights to this Reviewer and reserves the right to produce and distribute this Reviewer for commercial gain.

No Affiliation

The Reviewer is not affiliated with, endorsed by, or sponsored by any official testing organization, exam body, or educational institution. All references to the official examination are for identification purposes only and are not intended to imply any connection to or endorsement by the official exam bodies.

Contents

Chapter One

How to prepare the Examination Day

Active Study Techniques:

- Engage in active study techniques like teaching concepts to someone else, participating in study groups, or creating mind maps to deepen understanding and retention.

2. Set Clear Goals:

- Before studying, set clear, achievable goals for each study session, focusing on understanding rather than memorization.

3. Breaks and Rest:

- Use study techniques like the Pomodoro Technique to incorporate regular breaks, aiding concentration and preventing burnout. Also, ensure you get sufficient sleep in the days leading up to the exam.

4. Positive Affirmations:

- Reinforce your confidence and reduce anxiety with positive affirmations and visualization techniques.

5. Mock Exams:

- Regularly take timed practice exams under exam conditions to become familiar with the format and improve time management skills.

6. Healthy Snacks:

- Pack some healthy snacks, like nuts or fruits, to maintain energy levels during long exams.

7. Ergonomics:

- Ensure your chair and desk are comfortable and reduce strain. Good posture can also help with concentration.

8. Mnemonic Devices:

- Create and use mnemonic devices or acronyms to help remember complex concepts or lists.

9. Clarify Doubts:

- Before the exam day, clarify any doubts or areas of uncertainty with teachers or classmates.

10. Revision Plan:

- A few days before the exam, create a revision plan to review all topics, giving more time to weak areas.

11. Stay Informed:

- Know the exam's format, location, allowed materials, and start time. Avoid surprises on exam day.

12. Supportive Environment:

- Surround yourself with supportive and positive individuals who encourage your goals and understand the importance of your study time.

13. Mindfulness and Relaxation Techniques:

- Engage in mindfulness exercises or yoga to maintain focus and reduce stress.

14. Note Organization:

- Well-organized notes can save a lot of time during revision and help in quickly recalling concepts.

15. Realistic Expectations:

- Set achievable goals and realistic expectations to avoid undue stress.

16. Feedback Loop:

- After the exam, review your performance, focusing on both strengths and areas for improvement, and adjust your study strategies accordingly for future exams.

17. Stay Active:

- Regular physical activity can help in reducing stress and improving cognitive function.

18. Hydration:

- Drink adequate water throughout your study sessions and on the day of the exam to stay hydrated, as dehydration can impair cognitive function.

Chapter Two

Strategies for tackling multiple-choice questions

S trategies for tackling multiple-choice questions, here are additional general tips that can help you in taking exams:

1. Review and Practice Regularly:

- Regular review and practice of material lead to better retention and understanding. Use varied materials like flashcards, quizzes, and practice tests to reinforce learning.

2. Time Management:

- Start with easier questions to build confidence, and then tackle more difficult ones. Allocate time according to the marks allocated to a question, and don't exceed that time.

3. Understand the Question:

- Read every question carefully. Misreading a question can lead to unnecessary mistakes. If permitted, underline or highlight key terms in the questions.

4. Break Problems Down:

- For complex problems or essays, break them down into smaller, manageable parts and address each part methodically.

5. Use All Available Time:

- If you finish early, don't leave. Review your answers and make sure you didn't make any careless mistakes.

6. Stay Calm:

- Practice relaxation techniques like deep breathing or visualization to stay calm. Stress can hinder your ability to think clearly.

7. Skip and Return:

- If you get stuck on a question, don't spend too much time on it. Move on to the next and come back to it later if time allows.

8. Write Legibly:

- If the examiner can't read your writing, you might lose marks. So ensure that your handwriting is neat and legible.

9. Double-Check Your Work:

- Before submitting, review your work to catch any errors or incomplete answers. It's easy to make simple mistakes in a test situation.

10. Organize Your Thoughts:

- Before diving into answering an essay question, take a few minutes to jot down your thoughts and organize them cohesively.

11. Eat a Balanced Meal:

- Before the exam, eat a balanced meal to ensure you have

enough energy. Avoid heavy meals that can make you feel sluggish.

12. Hydrate:

- Stay hydrated, but be cautious not to drink excessive amounts right before the exam to avoid needing frequent bathroom breaks.

13. Arrive Early:

- Get to the exam venue a bit early to settle in and relax before the exam starts. Avoid discussing with peers right before the exam as it might increase anxiety.

14. Plan for the Unexpected:

- Bring extra pens, pencils, a watch, etc. Be prepared for any unforeseen circumstances that may occur during the exam.

15. Follow Instructions:

- Pay close attention to the instructions given, including time limits, and adhere strictly to them.

16. Healthy Lifestyle:

- Regular exercise, balanced nutrition, and adequate sleep play a crucial role in maintaining cognitive function and reducing anxiety.

Applying these strategies can significantly enhance your performance and reduce anxiety during exams. Balancing preparation and relaxation are key to maintaining optimum performance levels.

Chapter Three

Questions

1 .Q: What is the primary function of the respiratory system?

   a) Remove waste products

b) Transport nutrients

c) Oxygenate blood

d) Regulate body temperature

2.Q: Which of the following medications is an antipyretic?

a) Acetaminophen

b) Furosemide

c) Atorvastatin

d) Lisinopril

3.Q: A client with hypertension should be advised to restrict intake of which mineral?

a) Calcium

b) Potassium

c) Sodium

d) Magnesium

4.Q: Which of the following assessments is crucial for a geriatric patient experiencing confusion?

a) Mobility assessment

b) Nutritional status

c) Skin integrity

d) Hydration status

5.Q: A patient diagnosed with schizophrenia is experiencing auditory hallucinations. The initial nursing intervention should be to:

a) Administer antipsychotic medication as ordered.

b) Place the patient in seclusion.

c) Use therapeutic communication to discuss the hallucinations.

d) Restrict visitors to reduce stimulation.

6.Q: An elderly patient is at risk for skin breakdown. Which nursing intervention is the priority?

a) Applying moisturizers regularly

b) Repositioning the patient every 2 hours

c) Keeping the patient's skin dry and clean

d) Encouraging a high-protein diet

7.Q: A newborn's APGAR score at 1 minute is 7. The nurse should:

a) Administer oxygen immediately

b) Continue to monitor the newborn

c) Initiate CPR

d) Prepare for intubation

8.Q: Which infection control precaution is most effective in preventing the transmission of Clostridium difficile?

a) Hand hygiene with alcohol-based hand rub

b) Use of gloves and gowns

c) Airborne precautions

d) Handwashing with soap and water

9. Q: Which is a typical sign of a fracture?

a) Bruising

b) Crepitation

c) Cyanosis

d) Pallor

10. Q: A client is exhibiting Kussmaul respirations. The nurse understands this may be indicative of:

a) Pain

b) Hypoxia

c) Metabolic acidosis

d) Anxiety

11. Q: Which is the priority nursing intervention for a patient during a seizure?

a) Maintain an open airway

b) Administer antiseizure medication

c) Restrain the patient

d) Insert an oral airway

12. Q: What type of precaution is needed for a patient with pulmonary tuberculosis?

a) Contact

b) Droplet

c) Airborne

d) Standard

13. Q: What is a normal side effect of furosemide (Lasix)?

a) Hypokalemia

b) Hyperkalemia

c) Hypoglycemia

d) Hyperglycemia

14. Q: When assessing a patient with suspected dehydration, which of the following would be an expected finding?

a) Hypotension

b) Tachycardia

c) Decreased urine output

d) All of the above

15. Q: What is the priority nursing intervention for a client experiencing hypoglycemia?

a) Administer insulin

b) Provide carbohydrates

c) Administer glucagon

d) Start IV fluids

16. Q: A patient diagnosed with bipolar disorder is exhibiting signs of mania. Which of the following is a priority nursing intervention?

a) Encourage group therapy

b) Provide a quiet, low-stimulus environment

c) Encourage the exploration of feelings

d) Offer high-calorie, high-protein snacks

17. Q: The nurse is performing a neurological assessment. Which assessment finding would be of most concern?

a) Glasgow Coma Scale of 15

b) Pupils equal, round, and reactive to light

c) Decorticate posturing

d) Oriented to person, place, and time

18. Q: Which electrolyte imbalance is most likely in a patient with prolonged vomiting?

a) Hypernatremia

b) Hyponatremia

c) Hyperkalemia

d) Hypercalcemia

19. Q: A nurse is assessing a client with a suspected urinary tract infection (UTI). Which symptom would support this diagnosis?

a) Polyuria

b) Hematuria

c) Anuria

d) Oliguria

20. Q: Which of the following is a priority nursing intervention for a patient with a suspected stroke?

a) Administering antihypertensive medication

b) Elevating the head of the bed

c) Initiating a swallowing evaluation

d) Administering anticoagulant medication

21. Q: Which type of wound healing occurs when wound edges are not approximated?

   a) Primary intention

   b) Secondary intention

   c) Tertiary intention

   d) Quaternary intention

22. Q: In which condition is paradoxical chest movement a clinical feature?

   a) Asthma

   b) Pneumonia

   c) Flail chest

   d) Pulmonary embolism

23. Q: Which of the following dietary selections would be appropriate for a client with gout?

   a) Liver and onions

   b) Sardines on toast

   c) Grilled chicken salad

   d) Spinach and bacon salad

24. Q: Which nursing action is appropriate for a client with acute pancreatitis?

   a) Encourage frequent small meals.

   b) Place the client in a supine position.

   c) Encourage deep breathing and coughing exercises.

   d) Administer morphine for pain as needed.

25. Q: Which intervention is a priority for a client in the first hour following a burn injury?

a) Applying topical antibiotic ointment

b) Administering intravenous pain medication

c) Establishing intravenous access for fluid replacement

d) Administering tetanus prophylaxis

26. Q: The nurse is planning care for a client with delirium due to a urinary tract infection. Which intervention is the priority?

a) Orient the client frequently to time, place, and person.

b) Encourage family to bring in familiar items from home.

c) Administer antipsychotic medication as ordered.

d) Administer antibiotic medication as ordered.

27. Q: Which assessment is a priority for a client receiving heparin therapy?

a) Blood pressure

b) Respiratory rate

c) Activated partial thromboplastin time (aPTT)

d) Serum potassium level

28. Q: Which nursing action is most appropriate for a client experiencing an anaphylactic reaction?

a) Administer antihistamine medication as ordered.

b) Administer epinephrine as ordered.

c) Place the client in a high Fowler's position.

d) Start an IV with a large-bore needle.

29. Q: The nurse is caring for a client with chronic obstructive pulmonary disease (COPD). Which is an appropriate goal?

a) The client will have a respiratory rate of 30 breaths/min or less.

b) The client will have oxygen saturation levels above 95%.

c) The client will be free of dyspnea at rest.

d) The client will have clear lung sounds in all lobes.

30. Q: What would be a priority nursing intervention for a patient at risk of deep vein thrombosis?

   a) Encourage mobility

   b) Apply warm compresses

   c) Administer anti-inflammatory medication

   d) Elevate the legs

31. Q: Which of the following is the most appropriate intervention for a patient exhibiting signs of shock?

   a) Elevate the legs

   b) Administer a diuretic

   c) Encourage deep breathing exercises

   d) Provide a warm blanket

32. Q: Which of the following interventions is crucial for a patient suspected of having a myocardial infarction?

   a) Administer morphine

   b) Perform a 12-lead ECG

   c) Initiate IV access

   d) Administer aspirin

33. Q: A patient is diagnosed with congestive heart failure (CHF). What dietary advice should be given to this patient?

   a) High potassium, low sodium

   b) High protein, low fat

   c) High carbohydrate, low protein

   d) High fat, low carbohydrate

34. Q: A client with a history of seizures is prescribed phenytoin. Which lab value should the nurse monitor closely?

a) Sodium level

b) Potassium level

c) Blood glucose level

d) Serum phenytoin level

35. Q: The nurse is caring for a patient who has been vomiting for two days. Which of the following is a priority assessment?

a) Skin turgor

b) Bowel sounds

c) Pupil reaction

d) Reflexes

36. Q: A patient with end-stage renal disease is most at risk for developing which electrolyte imbalance?

a) Hypocalcemia

b) Hyponatremia

c) Hyperkalemia

d) Hypokalemia

37. Q: What is the priority intervention for a patient diagnosed with a flail chest?

a) Administer pain medication

b) Administer oxygen therapy

c) Apply a chest binder

d) Insert a chest tube

38. Q: Which of the following is a common side effect of opioid analgesics?

a) Diarrhea

b) Tachycardia

c) Hypertension

d) Constipation

39. Q: Which vaccine is contraindicated in a patient with a severe egg allergy?

a) Hepatitis B

b) Influenza

c) Tetanus

d) Pneumococcal

40. Q: A patient with a suspected upper GI bleed has a decreased hematocrit. The nurse understands this is due to:

a) Hemodilution

b) Hemolysis

c) Hemoconcentration

d) Hemorrhage

41. Q: For a patient with suspected meningitis, what is the priority nursing action?

a) Administering antibiotics

b) Performing a lumbar puncture

c) Isolating the patient

d) Administering antipyretics

42. Q: A nurse is caring for a patient with acute glomerulonephritis. Which of the following dietary selections is most appropriate?

a) High sodium and high protein

b) Low sodium and low protein

c) High potassium and high carbohydrate

d) Low potassium and high fat

43. Q: Which of the following is the best indicator of overall kidney function?

a) Blood urea nitrogen (BUN)

b) Serum creatinine

c) Urine specific gravity

d) Serum potassium

44. Q: A patient with rheumatoid arthritis (RA) complains of joint pain. Which type of medication will likely be ordered to address this complaint?

a) Antibiotic

b) Diuretic

c) Nonsteroidal anti-inflammatory drug (NSAID)

d) Antipyretic

45. Q: What is a potential complication of a fracture that requires immediate medical intervention?

a) Compartment syndrome

b) Infection

c) Delayed union

d) Avascular necrosis

46. Q: Which type of precautions should be implemented for a patient with a Clostridium difficile infection?

a) Droplet precautions

b) Airborne precautions

c) Contact precautions

d) Standard precautions

47. Q: For a client with hypothyroidism, which dietary choice is most appropriate?

a) High fiber and low calorie

b) High carbohydrate and high protein

c) Low fiber and high calorie

d) Low protein and high fat

48. Q: When providing tracheostomy care, which action is most important?

a) Suctioning the tracheostomy before cleaning

b) Cleaning the stoma site with hydrogen peroxide

c) Replacing the tracheostomy tube if it becomes dislodged

d) Keeping a spare tracheostomy tube at the bedside

49. Q: The nurse is teaching a patient with diabetes mellitus about foot care. Which statement by the patient indicates a need for further teaching?

a) "I will inspect my feet daily for any cuts or blisters."

b) "I will wear cotton socks and well-fitting shoes."

c) "I can use a heating pad on my feet to increase circulation."

d) "I will not walk barefoot, even indoors."

50. Q: What intervention is essential for a patient at risk of aspiration?

a) Elevate head of the bed to 45 degrees

b) Encourage coughing and deep breathing

c) Administer oxygen therapy

d) Encourage fluid intake

51. Q: Which of the following lab values would indicate impaired liver function?

a) Decreased albumin

b) Increased sodium

c) Decreased potassium

d) Increased calcium

52. Q: A nurse is educating a patient with gastroesophageal reflux disease (GERD). Which dietary choice should the patient avoid?

a) Grilled chicken

b) Spaghetti with tomato sauce

c) Baked potato

d) Steamed vegetables

53. Q: What intervention is vital for a patient diagnosed with a detached retina?

a) Administer eye drops

b) Place in a prone position

c) Apply a warm compress

d) Maintain strict bed rest

54. Q: Which clinical manifestation is a late sign of increased intracranial pressure (ICP)?

a) Nausea

b) Decreased level of consciousness

c) Headache

d) Pupillary asymmetry

55. Q: Which of the following drugs should be avoided in a patient with a history of asthma?

  a) Acetaminophen

  b) Aspirin

  c) Loratadine

  d) Dextromethorphan

56. Q: A nurse is monitoring a patient following a thyroidectomy. What complication requires immediate intervention?

  a) Stridor

  b) Hypocalcemia

  c) Hoarseness

  d) Neck swelling

57. Q: A patient with pneumonia is receiving antibiotic therapy. What is the best indicator that the treatment is effective?

  a) Normalized white blood cell count

  b) Clear lung sounds

  c) Decreased respiratory rate

  d) Normalized body temperature

58. Q: For a client with congestive heart failure, which assessment finding would indicate worsening condition?

  a) Decreased peripheral edema

  b) Increased urine output

  c) Weight gain

  d) Decreased respiratory rate

59. Q: What is a primary nursing consideration when caring for a patient receiving a blood transfusion?

a) Monitoring for hypotension

b) Administering with dextrose solution

c) Monitoring for a transfusion reaction

d) Administering a diuretic post-transfusion

60. Q: Which of the following findings is typical for a patient with Cushing's syndrome?

a) Hypotension

b) Hypoglycemia

c) Truncal obesity

d) Muscle wasting

61. Q: What is the most important nursing intervention for a patient with Myasthenia Gravis experiencing a myasthenic crisis?

a) Administering cholinesterase inhibitors

b) Initiating mechanical ventilation

c) Administering immunosuppressive agents

d) Monitoring vital capacity

62. Q: For a patient with a history of chronic obstructive pulmonary disease (COPD), which of the following would indicate acute respiratory distress?

a) Decreased respiratory rate

b) Decreased use of accessory muscles

c) Increased oxygen saturation

d) Pursed-lip breathing

63. Q: A patient is experiencing an acute asthma attack. What medication should the nurse prepare to administer?

a) Albuterol

b) Montelukast

c) Fluticasone

d) Salmeterol

64. Q: A patient is admitted with suspected meningitis. Which of the following is a priority nursing intervention?

a) Administer antibiotics immediately

b) Obtain blood cultures

c) Perform a neurologic assessment

d) Administer antipyretics

65. Q: Which medication should be administered to a patient experiencing an anaphylactic reaction?

a) Diphenhydramine

b) Epinephrine

c) Albuterol

d) Hydrocortisone

66. Q: For a patient with a spinal cord injury, what is a significant complication to monitor for?

a) Neurogenic shock

b) Increased intracranial pressure

c) Hemorrhagic shock

d) Pulmonary embolism

67. Q: A nurse is caring for a patient with a new colostomy. What is the priority nursing intervention?

a) Assessing stoma viability

b) Teaching about dietary restrictions

c) Encouraging fluid intake

d) Managing pain

68. Q: A patient with acute kidney injury (AKI) has a high potassium level. Which medication should the nurse anticipate administering?

a) Furosemide

b) Kayexalate

c) Sodium bicarbonate

d) Calcium gluconate

69. Q: What is a major complication associated with abrupt discontinuation of corticosteroid therapy?

a) Hyperglycemia

b) Adrenal crisis

c) Cushing's syndrome

d) Hypertension

70. Q: A patient with Crohn's disease would benefit most from which type of diet?

a) High fiber, low fat

b) High protein, low residue

c) Low carbohydrate, high fat

d) High calorie, low protein

71. Q: A patient has a burn injury affecting the entire depth of the skin but not underlying tissues. This burn is classified as:

a) Superficial

b) Superficial partial-thickness

c) Deep partial-thickness

d) Full-thickness

72. Q: Which is a common complication in patients with uncontrolled diabetes mellitus?

a) Hypoglycemia

b) Hypotension

c) Diabetic ketoacidosis

d) Respiratory alkalosis

73. Q: For a patient with a deep vein thrombosis (DVT), which medication should be administered as initial treatment?

a) Warfarin

b) Aspirin

c) Heparin

d) Clopidogrel

74. Q: A patient with acute pancreatitis should be positioned in which of the following ways to decrease pain?

a) Supine with legs elevated

b) Prone with head elevated

c) Left lateral decubitus

d) Fowler's position

75. Q: Which of the following is a potential side effect of doxorubicin, an antineoplastic medication?

a) Cardiotoxicity

b) Hypoglycemia

c) Hyperkalemia

d) Constipation

76. Q: A patient with acute glaucoma should avoid which class of medications?

a) Beta-blockers

b) Mydriatics

c) Carbonic anhydrase inhibitors

d) Prostaglandin analogs

77. Q: For a patient with a fractured hip, which type of surgical intervention is typically performed?

a) Arthroscopy

b) Hip arthroplasty

c) Lumbar laminectomy

d) Bone grafting

78. Q: A patient with tuberculosis (TB) should be placed in which type of isolation?

a) Droplet

b) Airborne

c) Contact

d) Protective

79. Q: Which assessment finding in a patient with cirrhosis indicates the presence of hepatic encephalopathy?

a) Asterixis

b) Ascites

c) Spider angiomas

d) Palmar erythema

80. Q: Which electrolyte imbalance is a common side effect of furosemide?

a) Hypercalcemia

b) Hyperkalemia

c) Hypomagnesemia

d) Hyponatremia

81. Q: In which type of shock is the administration of antihistamines most appropriate?

a) Cardiogenic shock

b) Anaphylactic shock

c) Septic shock

d) Hypovolemic shock

82. Q: A patient with hyperthyroidism is at risk for which of the following cardiovascular issues?

a) Bradycardia

b) Hypotension

c) Atrial fibrillation

d) Decreased cardiac output

83. Q: Which intervention is critical for a patient with Guillain-Barré syndrome?

a) Cardiac monitoring

b) Respiratory support

c) Seizure precautions

d) Pain management

84. Q: A patient with multiple sclerosis is experiencing muscle spasticity. Which medication is commonly used to manage this symptom?

   a) Baclofen

   b) Prednisone

   c) Interferon beta-1a

   d) Glatiramer acetate

85. Q: Which clinical manifestation is common in patients with rheumatoid arthritis?

   a) Hyperuricemia

   b) Morning stiffness

   c) Subcutaneous nodules

   d) Bone spur formation

86. Q: A patient with a brain tumor is exhibiting signs of increased intracranial pressure (ICP). Which medication is administered to decrease ICP?

   a) Mannitol

   b) Dexamethasone

   c) Phenobarbital

   d) Morphine

87. Q: Which is a priority nursing intervention for a patient who has just returned from having a bronchoscopy?

   a) Administering prescribed antibiotics

   b) Monitoring oxygen saturation levels

   c) Encouraging deep breathing exercises

   d) Assessing for the return of the gag reflex

88. Q: A patient with Addison's disease would primarily benefit from which type of therapy?

a) Insulin therapy

b) Hormone replacement therapy

c) Antihypertensive therapy

d) Diuretic therapy

89. Q: What condition is indicated by a sudden drop in hematocrit in a patient with a burn injury?

a) Hemolysis

b) Hemorrhage

c) Fluid shift

d) Infection

90. Q: Which medication is used as a first-line treatment for a patient with newly diagnosed hypertension?

a) Atenolol

b) Clonidine

c) Hydrochlorothiazide

d) Nifedipine

91. Q: Which assessment finding would be expected in a patient with acute pericarditis?

a) Pulsus paradoxus

b) Pericardial friction rub

c) Muffled heart sounds

d) Widened pulse pressure

92. Q: What is a common complication of long-term opioid use for chronic pain management?

a) Hyperalgesia

b) Tolerance

c) Dependence

d) Addiction

93. Q: A patient with osteoarthritis is scheduled for a total knee replacement. What is the priority preoperative teaching?

a) Use of assistive devices

b) Pain management

c) Physical therapy exercises

d) Wound care

94. Q: Which type of isolation is necessary for a patient with Clostridioides difficile (C. diff) infection?

a) Airborne

b) Droplet

c) Contact

d) Protective

95. Q: What is a characteristic feature of Parkinson's disease?

a) Hyperreflexia

b) Resting tremor

c) Spasticity

d) Rapid eye movement (REM) sleep behavior disorder

96. Q: Which of the following is a priority intervention for a patient with hypovolemic shock?

a) Administering antibiotics

b) Fluid resuscitation

c) Pain management

d) Administering vasopressors

97. Q: A patient with myasthenia gravis is at risk for which of the following complications?
a) Respiratory failure
b) Renal failure
c) Liver failure
d) Heart failure

98. Q: Which assessment finding indicates potential hypoxia in a postoperative patient?
a) Bradycardia
b) Hypertension
c) Restlessness
d) Hypothermia

99. Q: A patient with sepsis has a low blood pressure unresponsive to fluid resuscitation. Which medication is indicated in this scenario?
a) Dobutamine
b) Norepinephrine
c) Amiodarone
d) Furosemide

100. Q: A patient with an abdominal aortic aneurysm is at highest risk for which of the following complications?
a) Rupture
b) Thrombosis
c) Embolization
d) Dissection

101. Q: Which of the following interventions is important for a patient diagnosed with congestive heart failure (CHF)?

a) Fluid restriction

b) High-sodium diet

c) Fluid overload

d) High-potassium diet

102. Q: Which type of insulin has the quickest onset of action?

a) Regular insulin

b) NPH insulin

c) Insulin glargine

d) Insulin lispro

103. Q: What type of fracture is characterized by a bone fragment pulled off by a tendon or ligament?

a) Oblique

b) Avulsion

c) Comminuted

d) Spiral

104. Q: Which term describes the inability to recognize familiar objects or people?

a) Apraxia

b) Agnosia

c) Anomia

d) Aphasia

105. Q: Which action is most appropriate for a patient diagnosed with Cushing's syndrome?

a) Restricting fluids

b) Administering corticosteroids

c) Monitoring blood glucose levels

d) Administering antithyroid medications

106. Q: Which type of seizure is characterized by a brief loss of consciousness and staring spells?

a) Tonic-clonic

b) Absence

c) Myoclonic

d) Atonic

107. Q: A patient with suspected meningitis exhibits neck rigidity and involuntary hip and knee flexion when the neck is flexed. This sign is known as:

a) Kernig's sign

b) Brudzinski's sign

c) Babinski sign

d) McBurney's sign

108. Q: For a patient with asthma, which medication is used for quick relief of acute symptoms?

a) Montelukast

b) Albuterol

c) Fluticasone

d) Salmeterol

109. Q: Which of the following best describes the pain associated with a duodenal ulcer?

a) Sudden, sharp, and severe

b) Burning and cramp-like, relieved by eating

c) Gradual, dull, and achy, aggravated by eating

d) Intermittent, stabbing, and radiating to the back

110. Q: Which part of the brain is responsible for regulating temperature, hunger, and thirst?

a) Cerebellum

b) Medulla oblongata

c) Hypothalamus

d) Pons

111. Q: Which of the following conditions is a risk factor for the development of deep vein thrombosis (DVT)?

a) Hyperactivity

b) Dehydration

c) Immobility

d) Hypertension

112. Q: Which intervention is most appropriate for a patient with a pulmonary embolism?

a) Administration of beta-blockers

b) Administration of anticoagulants

c) Encouraging deep breathing exercises

d) Administration of diuretics

113. Q: Which diagnostic test is used to confirm a diagnosis of a myocardial infarction (MI)?

a) Electrocardiogram (ECG)

b) Chest X-ray

c) Echocardiogram

d) Cardiac enzyme levels

114. Q: What is the priority intervention for a patient with acute renal failure?

a) Monitor fluid balance

b) Monitor blood glucose levels

c) Administer anti-hypertensive medications

d) Encourage high-protein diet

115. Q: A patient diagnosed with diverticulitis should avoid consuming which of the following?

a) High-fiber foods

b) Dairy products

c) Seeds and nuts

d) Lean meats

116. Q: Which clinical manifestation is commonly observed in a patient with hypocalcemia?

a) Tachycardia

b) Hyperreflexia

c) Muscle weakness

d) Constipation

117. Q: Which of the following medications is a common treatment for a patient with bipolar disorder?

a) Lithium

b) Sertraline

c) Risperidone

d) Methylphenidate

118. Q: What is a typical feature of a tension headache?

a) Pulsating pain on one side of the head

b) Band-like pain around the head

c) Sharp, stabbing pain in the eye area

d) Throbbing pain at the base of the skull

119. Q: Which of the following is a common complication associated with a radical mastectomy?

a) Hemorrhage

b) Lymphedema

c) Pulmonary embolism

d) Infection

120. Q: Which intervention is a priority for a patient experiencing alcohol withdrawal?

a) Administering benzodiazepines

b) Encouraging participation in group therapy

c) Administering antipsychotic medications

d) Restricting fluids to avoid fluid overload

121. Q: Which action is crucial when caring for a patient with a suspected stroke?

a) Performing a thorough neurological assessment

b) Starting cardiopulmonary resuscitation (CPR)

c) Administering aspirin to prevent clot formation

d) Transporting the patient to a stroke center immediately

122. Q: Which sign is indicative of a positive Romberg test?

a) Inability to touch the nose with eyes closed

b) Loss of balance when standing with feet together and eyes closed

c) Inability to walk heel-to-toe in a straight line

d) Uncoordinated movements when performing rapid alternating movements

123. Q: What type of diet is recommended for a patient with acute pancreatitis?

a) High-protein diet

b) Low-fat diet

c) High-carbohydrate diet

d) NPO (nothing by mouth)

124. Q: What is the primary purpose of administering a beta-blocker to a patient with heart failure?

a) To increase heart rate

b) To decrease blood pressure

c) To improve cardiac output

d) To decrease myocardial oxygen consumption

125. Q: Which of the following is a risk factor for osteoporosis?

a) High calcium intake

b) Regular weight-bearing exercise

c) Postmenopausal status

d) High vitamin D levels

126. Q: Which action is most appropriate when performing a sterile dressing change?

a) Wearing clean gloves to remove the old dressing

b) Touching only the edges of the sterile field

c) Using the same sterile gloves to apply the new dressing

d) Cleaning the wound from the center outward in a circular motion

127. Q: What condition is characterized by a decrease in all types of blood cells, including red blood cells, white blood cells, and platelets?

a) Leukemia

b) Pancytopenia

c) Thrombocytopenia

d) Anemia

128. Q: Which of the following is a primary concern related to a patient with burn injuries?

a) Infection

b) Hypothermia

c) Hypertension

d) Hyperkalemia

129. Q: Which of the following respiratory disorders is characterized by irreversible enlargement of the air spaces distal to the terminal bronchioles?

a) Asthma

b) Chronic bronchitis

c) Emphysema

d) Pulmonary fibrosis

130. Q: Which of the following conditions is associated with chronic alcohol abuse?

a) Hypoglycemia

b) Hyperkalemia

c) Cirrhosis

d) Hypocalcemia

131. Q: What medication is used to treat anaphylactic reactions?

a) Diphenhydramine

b) Albuterol

c) Epinephrine

d) Hydrocortisone

132. Q: Which of the following is a common manifestation of right-sided heart failure?

a) Pulmonary edema

b) Peripheral edema

c) Paroxysmal nocturnal dyspnea

d) Orthopnea

133. Q: Which intervention is appropriate for a patient diagnosed with benign prostatic hyperplasia (BPH)?

a) Restricting fluid intake

b) Administering alpha-blockers

c) Performing regular prostate massage

d) Administering anti-inflammatory medications

134. Q: Which electrolyte imbalance is a potential side effect of loop diuretics?

a) Hypercalcemia

b) Hyperkalemia

c) Hypokalemia

d) Hypernatremia

135. Q: Which sign is characteristic of hyperthyroidism?

a) Weight gain

b) Bradycardia

c) Heat intolerance

d) Constipation

136. Q: Which intervention is a priority for a patient in the acute phase of a sickle cell crisis?

a) Administering iron supplements

b) Encouraging ambulation

c) Providing adequate hydration

d) Administering vitamin B12 injections

137. Q: Which clinical manifestation is a classic sign of diabetic ketoacidosis (DKA)?

a) Hypoventilation

b) Hypoglycemia

c) Kussmaul respirations

d) Bradycardia

138. Q: What is a common complication associated with mechanical ventilation?

a) Pneumothorax

b) Pulmonary edema

c) Pleural effusion

d) Pulmonary embolism

139. Q: Which dietary intervention is important for a patient with gout?

a) Increasing intake of purine-rich foods

b) Increasing protein intake

c) Avoiding alcohol consumption

d) Increasing carbohydrate intake

140. Q: Which nursing intervention is essential for a patient receiving enteral nutrition?

a) Administering medications via the feeding tube without flushing

b) Elevating the head of the bed at least 30 degrees during feeding

c) Mixing medications with enteral formula for ease of administration

d) Checking gastric residual volume every 8 hours

141. Q: Which of the following laboratory values is a common finding in a patient with anorexia nervosa?

a) Elevated white blood cell count

b) Elevated blood urea nitrogen (BUN)

c) Low serum potassium

d) Elevated serum glucose

142. Q: Which action is important for reducing the risk of catheter-associated urinary tract infections?

a) Keeping the drainage bag elevated above the level of the bladder

b) Irrigating the catheter daily with an antiseptic solution

c) Emptying the drainage bag at least once per shift

d) Securing the catheter to the thigh with tape

143. Q: Which condition is characterized by difficulty in swallowing?

a) Dyspepsia

b) Dysphasia

c) Dysphagia

d) Dyspnea

144. Q: Which type of medication is commonly used to treat patients with generalized anxiety disorder (GAD)?

a) Antipsychotic medications

b) Antidepressant medications

c) Antipyretic medications

d) Antispasmodic medications

145. Q: What is the recommended treatment for a patient with acute decompensated heart failure exhibiting pulmonary edema?

a) Administering oral beta-blockers

b) Administering IV diuretics

c) Initiating chest physiotherapy

d) Administering subcutaneous insulin

146. Q: Which of the following is an early sign of increased intracranial pressure?

a) Hypertension

b) Bradycardia

c) Altered level of consciousness

d) Unequal pupil size

147. Q: Which clinical manifestation is indicative of left-sided heart failure?

a) Jugular vein distention

b) Ascites

c) Pulmonary congestion

d) Hepatomegaly

148. Q: Which intervention is recommended for a patient with venous insufficiency?

a) Applying heat to the affected extremity

b) Elevating the legs above the level of the heart

c) Encouraging prolonged sitting or standing

d) Administering anticoagulant medication

149. Q: Which medication is used to treat Parkinson's disease by increasing the level of dopamine in the brain?

a) Baclofen

b) Levodopa

c) Gabapentin

d) Phenobarbital

150. Q: What is the priority intervention for a patient who has ingested a corrosive poison?

a) Inducing vomiting

b) Administering activated charcoal

c) Diluting with milk or water

d) Administering a laxative

151. Q: What intervention is critical for a patient diagnosed with Myasthenia Gravis during a myasthenic crisis?

a) Administering Cholinergic drugs

b) Administering Anticholinergic drugs

c) Encouraging physical exercise

d) Restricting fluid intake

152. Q: What is a priority nursing intervention for a patient with a suspected pulmonary embolism?

a) Administering anticoagulants

b) Encouraging coughing and deep breathing

c) Administering bronchodilators

d) Positioning the patient flat in bed

153. Q: Which symptom is most indicative of hypoglycemia?

a) Polyuria

b) Diaphoresis

c) Polydipsia

d) Polyphagia

154. Q: Which assessment is most important for a patient diagnosed with glaucoma?

a) Hearing assessment

b) Visual field assessment

c) Taste assessment

d) Smell assessment

155. Q: What intervention is most important for preventing pressure ulcers in immobilized patients?

a) Keeping the patient dry and clean

b) Applying topical antibiotics to red areas

c) Massaging bony prominences

d) Using doughnut-type cushions

156. Q: Which assessment finding would be of most concern for a patient with a history of chronic obstructive pulmonary disease (COPD)?

a) Barrel chest

b) Clubbed fingers

c) Pursed-lip breathing

d) Altered level of consciousness

157. Q: Which of the following interventions is essential when caring for a patient with renal calculi?

a) Encouraging fluid restriction

b) Administering calcium supplements

c) Encouraging high-calcium diet

d) Straining all urine

158. Q: Which clinical manifestation is most indicative of a tension pneumothorax?

a) Decreased respiratory rate

b) Tracheal deviation to the unaffected side

c) Presence of breath sounds on the affected side

d) Decreased use of accessory muscles

159. Q: Which of the following is a late sign of hypoxia?

a) Cyanosis

b) Restlessness

c) Tachycardia

d) Hypertension

160. Q: What clinical manifestation is indicative of right-sided heart failure?

a) Crackles in the lungs

b) Ascites

c) Pulmonary edema

d) Pleural effusion

161. Q: What is the priority nursing intervention for a patient who has had a cerebrovascular accident (CVA) with right-sided weakness?

a) Initiating seizure precautions

b) Placing the patient in a prone position

c) Performing passive range-of-motion exercises to the right side

d) Maintaining NPO status until a swallow study can be performed

162. Q: Which symptom is indicative of the hyperosmolar hyperglycemic state (HHS)?

a) Rapid, deep respirations

b) Decreased urine output

c) Dehydration

d) Fruity breath odor

163. Q: What is a major risk factor for developing acute kidney injury?

a) Hypercalcemia

b) Hypotension

c) Hypokalemia

d) Hypoxia

164. Q: Which of the following is the most effective measure to prevent the spread of infection?

a) Wearing gloves at all times

b) Hand hygiene

c) Wearing masks

d) Administering antibiotics prophylactically

165. Q: What should the nurse include when providing education to a patient with pernicious anemia?

a) Importance of iron supplementation

b) Need for lifelong vitamin B12 injections

c) Benefits of a diet high in folic acid

d) Encouraging intake of vitamin C-rich foods

166. Q: Which intervention is a priority for a patient diagnosed with a hemorrhagic stroke?

a) Administering thrombolytic agents

b) Maintaining a patent airway

c) Encouraging ambulation

d) Monitoring blood glucose levels

167. Q: What clinical manifestation is common in patients with hypothyroidism?

a) Diarrhea

b) Insomnia

c) Weight loss

d) Fatigue

168. Q: Which of the following is a common side effect of opioid analgesics?

a) Tachycardia

b) Hypertension

c) Constipation

d) Insomnia

169. Q: Which electrolyte imbalance is a common complication of diuretic therapy?

a) Hypernatremia

b) Hypercalcemia

c) Hypokalemia

d) Hyperkalemia

170. Q: Which of the following conditions is a contraindication for the administration of a live vaccine?

a) Pregnancy

b) Diabetes mellitus

c) Hypertension

d) Gout

171. Q: What is the initial intervention for a patient experiencing a seizure?

a) Administering antipyretics

b) Positioning the patient on the side

c) Restraining the patient

d) Inserting an oral airway

172. Q: Which clinical manifestation is a common finding in patients with active tuberculosis?

a) Hemoptysis

b) Weight gain

c) Bradycardia

d) Hypertension

173. Q: Which of the following interventions is important for managing a patient with delirium?

a) Restraining the patient for safety

b) Keeping the room brightly lit at all times

c) Providing a quiet and calm environment

d) Encouraging the family to stay away from the patient

174. Q: Which of the following is a typical sign of digoxin toxicity?

a) Tachycardia

b) Hyperkalemia

c) Visual disturbances

d) Hypertension

175. Q: Which of the following laboratory values would indicate a therapeutic level of anticoagulation for a patient receiving warfarin?

a) PT 12 seconds

b) INR 2.5

c) aPTT 28 seconds

d) Platelet count 150,000/mm^3

176. Q: What is the priority nursing intervention for a patient with suspected meningitis?

a) Administering antipyretics

b) Performing a lumbar puncture

c) Initiating droplet precautions

d) Monitoring neurological status

Answer: c) Initiating droplet precautions

177. Q: Which of the following would be the best source of protein for a patient with liver cirrhosis?

a) Cheese

b) Eggs

c) Red meat

d) Vegetables

178. Q: What is the primary purpose of administering corticosteroids to a patient with Addison's disease?

a) To increase blood glucose levels

b) To replace deficient hormones

c) To suppress the immune system

d) To promote diuresis

179. Q: Which of the following is a common clinical manifestation of severe anemia?

a) Hypertension

b) Tachycardia

c) Polycythemia

d) Hypercalcemia

180. Q: What is the most effective way to prevent the transmission of HIV?

a) Regular hand hygiene

b) Use of condoms during sexual activity

c) Receiving vaccinations

d) Avoiding sharing personal items

181. Q: For a patient with chronic kidney disease, which dietary modification is most important?

a) Low protein

b) Low carbohydrate

c) High fat

d) High fiber

182. Q: Which intervention is the most appropriate for managing a patient with agitated behavior?

a) Using restraints

b) Providing a quiet and low-stimulus environment

c) Offering frequent high-calorie snacks

d) Encouraging participation in group activities

183. Q: What is the priority nursing intervention for a patient who has just undergone a thyroidectomy and is experiencing tingling around the mouth and muscle twitching?

   a) Administering calcium gluconate

   b) Administering insulin

   c) Monitoring blood pressure

   d) Monitoring blood glucose levels

184. Q: Which of the following actions is most important when caring for a patient in the immediate post-operative period after abdominal surgery?

   a) Encouraging ambulation

   b) Encouraging deep breathing and coughing

   c) Encouraging fluid intake

   d) Monitoring for signs of infection

185. Q: What is the most significant risk factor for the development of colorectal cancer?

   a) High-fiber diet

   b) History of peptic ulcer disease

   c) Family history of the disease

   d) Sedentary lifestyle

186. Q: Which of the following would be the most appropriate choice of intravenous fluid for a dehydrated patient?

   a) 5% Dextrose in Water

   b) Lactated Ringer's solution

   c) 0.45% Sodium Chloride

   d) 25% Albumin

187. Q: What is the primary goal of palliative care?

a) To cure the underlying disease

b) To provide comfort and support

c) To prolong life at any cost

d) To aggressively treat all symptoms

188. Q: Which of the following is a common manifestation of deep vein thrombosis (DVT)?

a) Warmth and redness at the site

b) Decreased circumference of the affected limb

c) Decreased temperature of the affected limb

d) Pallor of the affected limb

189. Q: Which electrolyte should be closely monitored in a patient receiving digoxin therapy?

a) Sodium

b) Calcium

c) Potassium

d) Magnesium

190. Q: Which intervention is most beneficial in preventing ventilator-associated pneumonia?

a) Frequent oral care

b) Placing the patient in Trendelenburg position

c) Administering prophylactic antibiotics

d) Keeping the patient deeply sedated

191. Q: Which assessment finding would be consistent with a diagnosis of left-sided heart failure?

a) Peripheral edema

b) Ascites

c) Crackles in the lungs

d) Jugular vein distention

192. Q: Which medication class is considered the first-line treatment for hypertension?

a) Beta-blockers

b) Diuretics

c) Calcium channel blockers

d) Angiotensin-converting enzyme (ACE) inhibitors

193. Q: Which of the following conditions would require contact precautions?

a) Influenza

b) Tuberculosis

c) Scabies

d) Pneumonia

194. Q: Which action is a priority for a patient with a chest tube that has been accidentally removed?

a) Clamping the tube

b) Covering the site with a sterile dressing taped on three sides

c) Administering pain medication

d) Applying a tourniquet above the site

195. Q: What is the most common cause of burn injuries in older adults?

a) Electrical burns

b) Chemical burns

c) Scalds from hot liquids

d) Flame burns

196. Q: What is the initial step in managing a patient with suspected carbon monoxide poisoning?

a) Administering 100% oxygen

b) Initiating IV fluid therapy

c) Administering activated charcoal

d) Performing gastric lavage

197. Q: Which of the following is a key sign of hypovolemic shock?

a) Bradycardia

b) Hypertension

c) Tachypnea

d) Bounding pulse

198. Q: Which of the following statements is correct regarding the administration of a blood transfusion?

a) The transfusion should be completed within 6 hours

b) Vital signs should be monitored every 30 minutes during the transfusion

c) The transfusion should be started slowly for the first 15 minutes

d) The patient should not receive any other IV fluids during the transfusion

199. Q: Which of the following is a common symptom of right-sided heart failure?

a) Pulmonary edema

b) Cough producing frothy sputum

c) Jugular vein distention

d) Decreased urine output

200. Q: What is a priority nursing intervention for a patient diagnosed with a pulmonary embolism?

a) Administering anticoagulant medications as ordered

b) Encouraging coughing and deep breathing

c) Administering diuretics as ordered

d) Positioning the patient in the high Fowler's position

201. Q: What is the primary nursing intervention for a patient diagnosed with a flail chest?

a) Administration of high-flow oxygen

b) Administration of analgesics

c) Application of a chest binder

d) Administration of intravenous fluids

202. Q: Which nursing intervention is most appropriate for a patient experiencing an acute asthma attack?

a) Administering beta-blockers promptly

b) Initiating chest physiotherapy

c) Administering short-acting beta-agonists

d) Encouraging deep-breathing exercises

203. Q: Which laboratory value is most indicative of renal function?

a) Serum albumin

b) Serum creatinine

c) Blood urea nitrogen (BUN)

d) Hematocrit

204. Q: What is the recommended position for a patient after a liver biopsy?

a) Left lateral position

b) Right lateral position

c) Supine position

d) Prone position

205. Q: Which of the following is a common side effect of opioid analgesics?

a) Diarrhea

b) Tachycardia

c) Constipation

d) Hypertension

206. Q: How should the nurse respond to a patient who is experiencing auditory hallucinations?

a) Ignore the behavior and continue with care.

b) Ask the patient what the voices are saying.

c) Inform the patient that the voices are not real.

d) Restrain the patient for safety.

207. Q: Which of the following is the primary treatment for a patient with type 1 diabetes mellitus?

a) Oral hypoglycemic agents

b) Insulin therapy

c) Dietary modification

d) Exercise regimen

208. Q: What intervention is crucial when caring for a patient with Cushing's syndrome?

a) Restricting fluid intake

b) Providing a low-sodium diet

c) Encouraging mobility

d) Administering glucose supplements

209. Q: What is the first-line treatment for a patient in ventricular fibrillation?

a) CPR

b) Defibrillation

c) Administration of amiodarone

d) Cardiac catheterization

210. Q: What is the most important nursing intervention for a patient with suspected stroke?

a) Administering aspirin immediately

b) Positioning the patient on their side

c) Obtaining a CT scan promptly

d) Monitoring blood pressure every 15 minutes

211. Q: What is a common cause of upper GI bleeding?

a) Gastric ulcer

b) Crohn's disease

c) Diverticulitis

d) Colorectal cancer

212. Q: What is the primary goal of therapeutic communication with a suicidal patient?

a) Persuading the patient not to attempt suicide

b) Offering solutions to the patient's problems

c) Establishing a trusting and supportive relationship

d) Encouraging the patient to express anger

213. Q: Which of the following dietary selections would be appropriate for a patient with gout?
   a) Liver
   b) Anchovies
   c) Lentils
   d) Spinach

214. Q: What nursing intervention is most appropriate for a patient experiencing alcohol withdrawal?
   a) Providing a quiet, dimly lit environment
   b) Encouraging participation in group therapy
   c) Administering stimulant medications
   d) Restraining the patient to prevent self-harm

215. Q: Which of the following would be the most appropriate initial intervention for a patient who has ingested a corrosive poison?
   a) Inducing vomiting
   b) Administering activated charcoal
   c) Diluting the poison with milk or water
   d) Administering an antidote immediately

216. Q: What is the primary symptom of a tension pneumothorax?
   a) Deviated trachea
   b) Decreased respiratory rate
   c) Bradycardia
   d) Hyperresonance on percussion

217. Q: Which assessment finding indicates that a nasogastric (NG) tube is in the correct position?

a) Ability to speak clearly

b) Return of gastric content upon aspiration

c) Absence of abdominal distention

d) Presence of bowel sounds

218. Q: What is the priority nursing intervention for a patient diagnosed with bulimia nervosa?

a) Monitoring during and after meals

b) Encouraging a high-fiber diet

c) Providing nutritional education

d) Administering antidepressant medications

219. Q: Which nursing intervention is most important for a patient receiving peritoneal dialysis?

a) Monitoring blood pressure every 15 minutes

b) Ensuring the dialysate is warmed before infusion

c) Administering insulin as prescribed

d) Encouraging a high-protein diet

220. Q: What is a typical clinical manifestation of rheumatoid arthritis?

a) Heberden's nodes

b) Symmetrical joint inflammation

c) Scoliosis

d) Crepitus

221. Q: Which of the following is the appropriate first action for a nurse who discovers fire in a patient's room?

a) Activate the fire alarm

b) Extinguish the fire

c) Evacuate the patient

d) Close the doors and windows

222. Q: What is the most appropriate nursing intervention for a patient with Myasthenia Gravis experiencing a myasthenic crisis?

a) Administering additional anticholinesterase medications

b) Encouraging rest and conserving energy

c) Performing chest physiotherapy

d) Administering intravenous immunoglobulin

223. Q: What is the most important nursing intervention for a patient with a chest tube?

a) Clamping the tube regularly to check for air leaks

b) Encouraging deep breathing and coughing

c) Maintaining the drainage system below chest level

d) Stripping the tubing to maintain patency

224. Q: What is the primary symptom of infective endocarditis?

a) Chest pain

b) Dyspnea

c) Fever

d) Palpitations

225. Q: Which of the following would be most appropriate for managing a patient with delirium due to a urinary tract infection?

a) Administering antipsychotic medications

b) Applying physical restraints

c) Treating the underlying infection

d) Providing sensory stimulation

226. Q: Which of the following is the most common cause of dementia in the elderly?

a) Huntington's disease

b) Creutzfeldt-Jakob disease

c) Alzheimer's disease

d) Multiple sclerosis

227. Q: Which of the following foods would be most appropriate for a patient with a history of kidney stones?

a) Spinach

b) Chocolate

c) Nuts

d) Rice

228. Q: Which of the following is a common side effect of radiation therapy?

a) Alopecia

b) Hypertension

c) Tachycardia

d) Hyperkalemia

229. Q: What is the priority nursing intervention for a patient experiencing an anaphylactic reaction?

a) Administering an antihistamine

b) Administering epinephrine

c) Starting an IV line

d) Administering a steroid

230. Q: Which of the following interventions is most important for preventing pressure ulcers in immobilized patients?

a) Applying talcum powder to reduce friction

b) Massaging bony prominences regularly

c) Changing the patient's position every two hours

d) Keeping the head of the bed elevated

231. Q: Which is a correct hand hygiene step when using hand sanitizer?

a) Washing hands with water after applying sanitizer

b) Drying hands with a towel after applying sanitizer

c) Rubbing hands together until the sanitizer is dry

d) Applying a small amount of sanitizer

232. Q: What is a critical nursing action when caring for a patient with a tracheostomy?

a) Suctioning the tracheostomy every hour

b) Changing the tracheostomy ties daily

c) Keeping a spare tracheostomy tube at the bedside

d) Providing oral care every 8 hours

233. Q: Which of the following is a key component in managing a patient with reactive hypoglycemia?

a) Encouraging a diet high in simple carbohydrates

b) Administering regular insulin as needed

c) Encouraging frequent, small meals

d) Administering oral hypoglycemic agents

234. Q: What is the appropriate intervention for a patient experiencing a sickle cell crisis?

a) Administration of iron supplements

b) High-dose vitamin C administration

c) Hydration and pain management

d) Blood transfusion

235. Q: What is a key nursing intervention for a patient diagnosed with Guillain-Barré Syndrome?

a) Encouraging physical therapy and mobility

b) Monitoring respiratory function and providing ventilatory support as needed

c) Administering steroids to reduce inflammation

d) Encouraging a high-protein diet

236. Q: What is the priority nursing intervention for a patient with hyperkalemia?

a) Administering sodium polystyrene sulfonate

b) Encouraging intake of potassium-rich foods

c) Administering IV calcium gluconate

d) Administering a loop diuretic

237. Q: Which of the following is the most accurate method for confirming the placement of a nasogastric tube?

a) Auscultating for a whooshing sound after injecting air

b) Observing the tube through the nostril to the stomach

c) Checking the pH of the aspirate

d) Observing for respiratory distress

238. Q: What is the most important factor in wound healing?

a) Age of the patient

b) Nutritional status

c) Presence of infection

d) Wound size

239. Q: Which medication would be most appropriate for a patient experiencing acute anxiety?

a) Diazepam

b) Fluoxetine

c) Lithium carbonate

d) Haloperidol

240. Q: Which of the following is a common sign of left-sided heart failure?

a) Jugular vein distention

b) Peripheral edema

c) Crackles in the lungs

d) Ascites

241. Q: Which of the following is a priority nursing intervention for a patient with a history of falls?

a) Encouraging the use of a walker or cane

b) Placing the bed in the lowest position

c) Encouraging the patient to rise quickly from a sitting position

d) Leaving the bedside commode at a distance to encourage mobility

242. Q: What is the most appropriate action for a nurse when a patient refuses medication?

a) Coercing the patient to take the medication

b) Documenting the refusal and notifying the healthcare provider

c) Administering the medication in a different form without informing the patient

d) Discarding the medication without documentation

243. Q: Which of the following would be most appropriate to include in the teaching plan for a patient with a new colostomy?
a) Avoiding all fruits and vegetables
b) Performing colostomy irrigations daily
c) Restricting fluid intake
d) Encouraging regular skin care around the stoma

244. Q: What should a nurse prioritize when caring for a patient with a seizure disorder who is experiencing a seizure?
a) Inserting an oral airway
b) Holding the patient down to prevent injury
c) Timing the duration of the seizure
d) Protecting the patient's head and maintaining airway patency

245. Q: Which of the following is a critical nursing action when administering a blood transfusion?
a) Starting the transfusion slowly and staying with the patient for the first 15 minutes
b) Running the blood transfusion at a fast rate to prevent clotting
c) Administering the blood transfusion with dextrose solution
d) Mixing medications in the blood transfusion bag

246. Q: Which of the following is the best indicator of fluid balance in a patient?
a) Blood pressure
b) Heart rate

c) Daily weight

d) Urine output

247. Q: Which of the following should a nurse monitor in a patient receiving heparin therapy?

a) Prothrombin time (PT)

b) International normalized ratio (INR)

c) Activated partial thromboplastin time (aPTT)

d) Hemoglobin

248. Q: Which of the following is a priority nursing action for a patient with an altered level of consciousness (ALOC)?

a) Monitoring vital signs every 4 hours

b) Placing the patient in a prone position

c) Maintaining a patent airway

d) Providing oral fluids

249. Q: When caring for a patient with glaucoma, what is an important teaching point the nurse should emphasize?

a) Administration of eye drops to reduce intraocular pressure

b) Encouraging regular eye examinations to change prescription glasses

c) Avoiding reading and other activities that strain the eyes

d) Informing the healthcare provider of any color vision changes

250. Q: What is the priority nursing intervention for a patient with myasthenia gravis experiencing a myasthenic crisis?

a) Administering cholinesterase inhibitors

b) Administering corticosteroids

c) Initiating mechanical ventilation

d) Administering intravenous immunoglobulin

251. Q: Which of the following is the most appropriate dietary recommendation for a patient with chronic kidney disease?
a) High-protein diet
b) Low-calcium diet
c) Low-potassium diet
d) High-phosphorus diet

252. Q: What is a key nursing intervention for a patient post-cardiac catheterization?
a) Encouraging ambulation immediately after the procedure
b) Monitoring the catheter insertion site for bleeding or hematoma formation
c) Allowing the patient to consume food and water immediately after the procedure
d) Positioning the patient with the head of the bed elevated 45 degrees

253. Q: What is the primary nursing intervention for a patient presenting with symptoms of a stroke?
a) Administering aspirin immediately
b) Performing a glucose check
c) Positioning the patient on their left side
d) Initiating antihypertensive therapy

254. Q: What would be a priority nursing intervention for a patient with suspected meningitis?
a) Administering antipyretics
b) Starting antibiotic therapy promptly after cultures are obtained

c) Encouraging fluid intake

d) Placing in a room with a positive pressure environment

255. Q: Which vitamin is essential for proper blood clotting?

a) Vitamin A

b) Vitamin D

c) Vitamin K

d) Vitamin E

256. Q: For a patient with a suspected pulmonary embolism, what is the priority intervention?

a) Administering oxygen

b) Administering anticoagulants

c) Encouraging ambulation

d) Providing pain relief

257. Q: What is the most critical intervention for a newborn with a suspected congenital heart defect?

a) Administering digoxin

b) Providing supplemental oxygen

c) Starting prophylactic antibiotics

d) Immediate surgical intervention

258. Q: What is a priority assessment for patients with chronic obstructive pulmonary disease (COPD)?

a) Pulse oximetry

b) Bowel sounds

c) Peripheral pulses

d) Skin turgor

259. Q: What is the first-line treatment for a patient presenting with diabetic ketoacidosis (DKA)?

a) Insulin therapy

b) Oral hypoglycemic agents

c) Bicarbonate administration

d) Intravenous fluids

260. Q: What is a priority nursing intervention for a patient with hypovolemic shock?

a) Administration of vasopressors

b) Administration of IV fluids

c) Placement in Trendelenburg position

d) Administration of blood products

261. Q: What is the appropriate intervention for a patient with a rectal temperature of 105°F (40.5°C)?

a) Applying warm compresses

b) Administering acetaminophen

c) Encouraging increased fluid intake

d) Providing additional blankets

262. Q: Which lab value is indicative of impaired kidney function?

a) Elevated serum creatinine

b) Decreased blood urea nitrogen (BUN)

c) Decreased white blood cell count

d) Elevated platelet count

263. Q: What is the priority nursing action for an unconscious patient?

a) Checking blood glucose levels

b) Performing a neurological exam

c) Establishing an IV line

d) Initiating CPR

264. Q: When caring for a patient with heart failure, which dietary modification is most appropriate?

a) High-protein diet

b) Low-sodium diet

c) High-carbohydrate diet

d) High-fat diet

265. Q: What is the most important nursing intervention for a patient who has undergone a total laryngectomy?

a) Teaching the patient how to speak using an artificial larynx

b) Managing pain effectively

c) Providing emotional support

d) Monitoring for signs of infection

266. Q: Which medication is used as a first-line treatment for hypertensive crisis?

a) Atenolol

b) Nitroprusside

c) Lisinopril

d) Hydrochlorothiazide

267. Q: What is the priority nursing action for a patient in ventricular fibrillation?

a) Administering amiodarone IV push

b) Starting cardiopulmonary resuscitation (CPR)

c) Defibrillation

d) Administering epinephrine IV push

268. Q: Which of the following is a critical intervention for a patient with acute respiratory distress syndrome (ARDS)?

a) Administering high-flow oxygen

b) Administering corticosteroids

c) Placing the patient in a prone position

d) Administering diuretics

269. Q: What intervention is crucial for a patient diagnosed with tuberculosis?

a) Administering a live vaccine

b) Placing the patient in airborne isolation

c) Administering broad-spectrum antibiotics

d) Performing a bronchoscopy

270. Q: For a patient with severe anemia, what is the priority nursing intervention?

a) Monitoring for signs of infection

b) Administering iron supplements

c) Encouraging increased fluid intake

d) Administering a blood transfusion

271. Q: Which action is most appropriate for a patient with a pulmonary embolism and hypotension?

a) Administering diuretics

b) Administering anticoagulants

c) Administering vasopressors

d) Encouraging deep-breathing exercises

272. Q: When caring for a patient with severe dehydration, what is the priority nursing intervention?

a) Monitoring intake and output

b) Encouraging oral fluid intake

c) Administering IV fluids

d) Monitoring for signs of overhydration

273. Q: Which intervention is most important for a patient with acute pancreatitis?

a) Administering pain medication

b) Encouraging a low-fat diet

c) Administering insulin

d) Placing the patient in a side-lying position

274. Q: What is the priority nursing action for a patient with an upper gastrointestinal bleed?

a) Starting an IV line

b) Administering a proton pump inhibitor

c) Inserting a nasogastric tube

d) Placing the patient in a semi-Fowler's position

275. Q: Which of the following interventions is most appropriate for a patient with a deep vein thrombosis (DVT)?

a) Encouraging ambulation

b) Applying warm compresses

c) Administering anticoagulants

d) Performing a massage at the site

276. Q: What is the primary intervention for a patient with acute glomerulonephritis?

a) Administering antibiotics

b) Administering antihypertensive medications

c) Monitoring urine output

d) Encouraging fluid intake

277. Q: Which of the following interventions is most important for a patient with a head injury?

a) Monitoring neurological status frequently

b) Administering pain medication

c) Encouraging cough and deep breathing exercises

d) Applying a cold compress to the head

278. Q: Which of the following is the priority nursing action for a patient with third-degree burns covering 30% of the body?

a) Administering intravenous fluids

b) Applying topical antibiotics

c) Debriding necrotic tissue

d) Administering pain medication

279. Q: Which of the following interventions is most crucial for a patient with suspected spinal injury?

a) Administering corticosteroids

b) Immobilizing the spine

c) Administering muscle relaxants

d) Performing a neurological assessment

280. Q: What is the priority nursing action for a patient experiencing an anaphylactic reaction?

a) Administering an antihistamine

b) Administering epinephrine

c) Administering a steroid

d) Administering a bronchodilator

281. Q: What is the priority nursing intervention for a patient with acute pericarditis?

a) Administering NSAIDs

b) Administering corticosteroids

c) Monitoring cardiac rhythms

d) Placing the patient in Fowler's position

282. Q: For a patient with chronic venous insufficiency, which of the following interventions is most appropriate?

a) Applying warm compresses

b) Encouraging leg elevation

c) Administering diuretics

d) Encouraging exercise

283. Q: Which medication should be administered immediately to a patient in status epilepticus?

a) Lorazepam (Ativan)

b) Phenobarbital

c) Phenytoin (Dilantin)

d) Valproic acid (Depakote)

284. Q: What is the priority nursing intervention for a patient with a flail chest?

a) Pain management

b) Administration of muscle relaxants

c) Assisted ventilation

d) Application of a chest binder

285. Q: What intervention is most crucial for a patient who has ingested a corrosive poison?

a) Administering activated charcoal

b) Inducing vomiting

c) Diluting the poison with milk or water

d) Administering an antidote

286. Q: Which intervention is most important for a patient diagnosed with Clostridium difficile infection?

a) Encouraging fluid intake

b) Administering probiotics

c) Placing in contact isolation

d) Administering antidiarrheal medications

287. Q: What is a priority intervention for a patient with myasthenia gravis experiencing a crisis?

a) Administering anticholinesterase medications

b) Implementing fall precautions

c) Administering corticosteroids

d) Providing respiratory support

288. Q: Which dietary modification is most appropriate for a patient with gallstones?

a) High-carbohydrate diet

b) Low-fat diet

c) High-protein diet

d) Low-sodium diet

Answer: b) Low-fat diet

289. Q: What is the primary nursing intervention for a patient experiencing a sickle cell crisis?

   a) Administering oxygen

   b) Administering pain medication

   c) Administering fluids

   d) Administering folic acid

290. Q: Which intervention is crucial for a patient with acute angle-closure glaucoma?

   a) Administering osmotic diuretics

   b) Administering anti-inflammatory medications

   c) Administering beta-blockers

   d) Performing eye exercises

291. Q: What is the priority nursing intervention for a patient with compartment syndrome?

   a) Elevating the affected limb

   b) Applying a compression bandage

   c) Administering anti-inflammatory medications

   d) Preparing the patient for fasciotomy

292. Q: Which nursing action is priority for a patient with a suspected bowel obstruction?

   a) Administering laxatives

   b) Administering antiemetic medications

   c) Initiating nasogastric suction

   d) Encouraging fluid intake

293. Q: Which of the following is a priority for a patient with a chest tube that has been accidentally removed?

a) Reinserting the chest tube immediately

b) Covering the site with a sterile dressing

c) Applying a tight, occlusive dressing to the site

d) Administering pain medication

294. Q: What is the priority nursing intervention for a patient in malignant hyperthermia?

a) Administering dantrolene

b) Applying cooling blankets

c) Administering antipyretics

d) Monitoring vital signs every 15 minutes

295. Q: Which of the following is the most appropriate intervention for a patient with Parkinson's disease experiencing bradykinesia?

a) Administering levodopa/carbidopa

b) Administering anticholinergic medications

c) Implementing a regular exercise program

d) Administering muscle relaxants

296. Q: What is the priority nursing intervention for a patient experiencing a hemorrhagic stroke?

a) Administering anticoagulant medications

b) Maintaining a patent airway

c) Administering thrombolytic agents

d) Monitoring blood pressure levels

297. Q: Which intervention is a priority for a patient with Bell's palsy?

a) Administering antiviral medications

b) Administering muscle relaxants

c) Providing eye protection

d) Implementing a soft diet

298. Q: What is the most appropriate nursing action for a patient with a suspected upper GI bleed?

a) Initiating a proton pump inhibitor

b) Administering oral iron supplements

c) Performing guaiac test on stools

d) Administering vitamin K

299. Q: What is the priority nursing action for a patient with Addison's disease experiencing a crisis?

a) Administering hydrocortisone

b) Monitoring blood glucose levels

c) Administering fludrocortisone

d) Encouraging a diet high in sodium

300. Q: Which intervention is critical for a patient with an acute myocardial infarction?

a) Administering nitroglycerin

b) Administering beta-blockers

c) Administering morphine sulfate

d) Administering aspirin

Chapter Four

Questions and Answers with Explanations

1 .Q: What is the primary function of the respiratory system?

a) Remove waste products

b) Transport nutrients

c) Oxygenate blood

d) Regulate body temperature

Answer: c) Oxygenate blood

Explanation:

The primary function of the respiratory system is to oxygenate blood. It achieves this by facilitating the exchange of oxygen and carbon dioxide between the atmosphere and the bloodstream through the process of respiration. Oxygen is essential for cellular metabolism, and the removal of carbon dioxide, a waste

2.Q: Which of the following medications is an antipyretic?

a) Acetaminophen

b) Furosemide

c) Atorvastatin

d) Lisinopril

Answer: a) Acetaminophen

Explanation:

Acetaminophen is a medication with antipyretic and analgesic properties, meaning it can reduce fever (antipyretic) and relieve pain (analgesic). It is not an anti-inflammatory agent, so it doesn't reduce inflammation. Furosemide is a diuretic, Atorvastatin is a statin used for lowering cholesterol, and Lisinopril is an ACE inhibitor used for managing hypertension.

3.Q: A client with hypertension should be advised to restrict intake of which mineral?

a) Calcium

b) Potassium

c) Sodium

d) Magnesium

Answer: c) Sodium

Explanation:

People with hypertension are often advised to restrict their intake of sodium. High sodium intake can lead to fluid retention, which can increase blood pressure. The other minerals listed—calcium, potassium, and magnesium—are generally not restricted in hypertension, and they play critical roles in maintaining optimal health. In some cases, adequate intake of potassium and magnesium is encouraged as they can help in the management of blood pressure.

4.Q: Which of the following assessments is crucial for a geriatric patient experiencing confusion?

a) Mobility assessment

b) Nutritional status

c) Skin integrity

d) Hydration status

Answer: d) Hydration status

Explanation:

For geriatric patients experiencing confusion, assessing hydration status is crucial. Dehydration is common in older adults and can lead to confusion, delirium, urinary tract infections, and other serious conditions. While all the assessments listed are important in geriatric care, in the context of sudden onset confusion, determining hydration status is particularly important to either rule out or confirm dehydration as a contributing factor.

5.Q: A patient diagnosed with schizophrenia is experiencing auditory hallucinations. The initial nursing intervention should be to:

a) Administer antipsychotic medication as ordered.

b) Place the patient in seclusion.

c) Use therapeutic communication to discuss the hallucinations.

d) Restrict visitors to reduce stimulation.

Answer: c) Use therapeutic communication to discuss the hallucinations.

Explanation:

When a patient is experiencing auditory hallucinations, using therapeutic communication to discuss the hallucinations is often the initial nursing intervention. This approach helps in validating the patient's experience, offering support, and gathering information about the hallucination's content and impact. While antipsychotic medication may be part of the management plan, the immediate response should be to engage the patient in a therapeutic manner. Seclusion and visitor restriction might be necessary in some cases but are not the initial interventions, especially before understanding the specific context and triggers of the hallucinations.

6.Q: An elderly patient is at risk for skin breakdown. Which nursing intervention is the priority?

a) Applying moisturizers regularly

b) Repositioning the patient every 2 hours

c) Keeping the patient's skin dry and clean

d) Encouraging a high-protein diet

Answer: b) Repositioning the patient every 2 hours

Explanation:

- For elderly patients, especially those with limited mobility, pressure ulcers or bedsores are a significant risk due to prolonged pressure on the skin, which limits blood flow to the skin, depriving it of nutrients and oxygen. Repositioning the patient every 2 hours is crucial in preventing skin breakdown by relieving pressure and improving blood flow to the skin.

- While keeping the skin dry and clean, applying moisturizers, and encouraging a high-protein diet are also important interventions to maintain skin integrity, repositioning is generally considered the priority intervention to directly address the risk of pressure ulcers in immobile or bedridden patients.

7.Q: A newborn's APGAR score at 1 minute is 7. The nurse should:

a) Administer oxygen immediately

b) Continue to monitor the newborn

c) Initiate CPR

d) Prepare for intubation

Answer: b) Continue to monitor the newborn

Explanation:

- The APGAR score is a quick evaluation tool for assessing the physical condition of a newborn immediately after birth at 1 minute and again at 5 minutes. The score ranges from 0 to 10, with 10 being the best possible condition. A score of 7 is considered fairly normal, indicating that the newborn is in fairly good condition but may require some medical attention. There is no indication for immediate oxygen administration, CPR, or intubation with an APGAR score of 7 at 1 minute. The appropriate nursing action would be to continue to monitor the newborn.

8.Q: Which infection control precaution is most effective in preventing the transmission of Clostridium difficile?

    a) Hand hygiene with alcohol-based hand rub

    b) Use of gloves and gowns

    c) Airborne precautions

    d) Handwashing with soap and water

Answer: d) Handwashing with soap and water

Explanation:

- Clostridium difficile is a bacterium that causes diarrhea and more serious intestinal conditions such as colitis. It is transmitted through spores that are not killed by alcohol-based hand rubs. Therefore, handwashing with soap and water is the most effective way to prevent the transmission of Clostridium difficile as it helps in removing the spores. The use of gloves and gowns is also important but handwashing with soap and water is the primary and most effective infection control precaution for Clostridium difficile.

9. Q: Which is a typical sign of a fracture?

a) Bruising

b) Crepitation

c) Cyanosis

d) Pallor

Answer: b) Crepitation

Explanation:

- Crepitation refers to the grating sound or feeling experienced when the broken ends of a bone move together. It is a typical sign of a fracture. While bruising, cyanosis, and pallor can be associated with fractures, they are not specific signs and can occur in various other conditions.

10. Q: A client is exhibiting Kussmaul respirations. The nurse understands this may be indicative of:

a) Pain

b) Hypoxia

c) Metabolic acidosis

d) Anxiety

Answer: c) Metabolic acidosis

Explanation:

- Kussmaul respirations are deep, rapid breaths that are characteristic of metabolic acidosis, particularly diabetic ketoacidosis (DKA). This breathing pattern is the body's attempt to reduce the acidity of the blood by expelling more carbon dioxide. Pain, hypoxia, and anxiety can cause changes in respiratory rate and pattern, but they are not specifically associated with Kussmaul respirations.

11. Q: Which is the priority nursing intervention for a patient during a seizure?

a) Maintain an open airway

b) Administer antiseizure medication

c) Restrain the patient

d) Insert an oral airway

Answer: a) Maintain an open airway

Explanation: During a seizure, maintaining an open airway is the priority to prevent hypoxia. The tongue or secretions can obstruct the airway, making it imperative to ensure that it remains clear.

12. Q: What type of precaution is needed for a patient with pulmonary tuberculosis?

a) Contact

b) Droplet

c) Airborne

d) Standard

Answer: c) Airborne

Explanation: Pulmonary tuberculosis is transmitted through the air, necessitating airborne precautions, including a negative pressure room and N95 masks for healthcare workers.

13. Q: What is a normal side effect of furosemide (Lasix)?

a) Hypokalemia

b) Hyperkalemia

c) Hypoglycemia

d) Hyperglycemia

Answer: a) Hypokalemia

Explanation: Furosemide (Lasix) can cause the loss of potassium, leading to hypokalemia. Monitoring potassium levels and supplementing as necessary are important when using this medication.

14. Q: When assessing a patient with suspected dehydration, which of the following would be an expected finding?

a) Hypotension

b) Tachycardia

c) Decreased urine output

d) All of the above

Answer: d) All of the above

Explanation: Dehydration can lead to hypotension, tachycardia, and decreased urine output as the body attempts to conserve fluid.

15. Q: What is the priority nursing intervention for a client experiencing hypoglycemia?

a) Administer insulin

b) Provide carbohydrates

c) Administer glucagon

d) Start IV fluids

Answer: b) Provide carbohydrates

Explanation: The priority intervention for hypoglycemia is to provide quick-acting carbohydrates to restore blood glucose levels, preventing further complications like loss of consciousness or seizures.

16. Q: A patient diagnosed with bipolar disorder is exhibiting signs of mania. Which of the following is a priority nursing intervention?

a) Encourage group therapy

b) Provide a quiet, low-stimulus environment

c) Encourage the exploration of feelings

d) Offer high-calorie, high-protein snacks

Answer: b) Provide a quiet, low-stimulus environment

Explanation: Patients experiencing mania are often overstimulated, and providing a low-stimulus environment can help in reducing agitation and promoting safety.

17. Q: The nurse is performing a neurological assessment. Which assessment finding would be of most concern?

a) Glasgow Coma Scale of 15

b) Pupils equal, round, and reactive to light

c) Decorticate posturing

d) Oriented to person, place, and time

Answer: c) Decorticate posturing

Explanation: Decorticate posturing is a sign of severe brain damage and is considered more concerning compared to normal findings or those suggesting an optimal level of neurological function, such as a Glasgow Coma Scale of 15 or being oriented to person, place, and time.

18. Q: Which electrolyte imbalance is most likely in a patient with prolonged vomiting?

a) Hypernatremia

b) Hyponatremia

c) Hyperkalemia

d) Hypercalcemia

Answer: b) Hyponatremia

Explanation: Prolonged vomiting can lead to a loss of sodium, causing hyponatremia, which can be life-threatening if not addressed.

19. Q: A nurse is assessing a client with a suspected urinary tract infection (UTI). Which symptom would support this diagnosis?

a) Polyuria

b) Hematuria

c) Anuria

d) Oliguria

Answer: b) Hematuria

Explanation: Hematuria or the presence of blood in the urine is a common symptom in UTIs, and it supports the diagnosis of a urinary tract infection.

20. Q: Which of the following is a priority nursing intervention for a patient with a suspected stroke?

a) Administering antihypertensive medication

b) Elevating the head of the bed

c) Initiating a swallowing evaluation

d) Administering anticoagulant medication

Answer: c) Initiating a swallowing evaluation

Explanation: In patients with suspected stroke, initiating a swallowing evaluation is crucial to prevent aspiration, which can lead to pneumonia.

21. Q: Which type of wound healing occurs when wound edges are not approximated?

a) Primary intention

b) Secondary intention

c) Tertiary intention

d) Quaternary intention

Answer: b) Secondary intention

Explanation: Secondary intention healing occurs when wound edges are not approximated, typically seen in larger, open wounds, ulcers, or wounds with tissue loss. Healing occurs from the base of the wound bed upwards and can take longer compared to primary intention, where wound edges are approximated, such as in surgical incisions.

22. Q: In which condition is paradoxical chest movement a clinical feature?

a) Asthma

b) Pneumonia

c) Flail chest

d) Pulmonary embolism

Answer: c) Flail chest

Explanation: Paradoxical chest movement is seen in flail chest, a condition where a segment of the rib cage is detached from the rest of the chest wall, usually due to trauma. This detached segment moves in the opposite direction to the rest of the chest wall during respiration, creating paradoxical movement.

23. Q: Which of the following dietary selections would be appropriate for a client with gout?

   a) Liver and onions

   b) Sardines on toast

   c) Grilled chicken salad

   d) Spinach and bacon salad

   Answer: c) Grilled chicken salad

Explanation: Individuals with gout are advised to avoid foods high in purines like organ meats (liver) and certain fish (sardines). Grilled chicken salad is a lower-purine option.

24. Q: Which nursing action is appropriate for a client with acute pancreatitis?

   a) Encourage frequent small meals.

   b) Place the client in a supine position.

   c) Encourage deep breathing and coughing exercises.

   d) Administer morphine for pain as needed.

   Answer: c) Encourage deep breathing and coughing exercises.

Explanation: For acute pancreatitis, it is essential to maintain lung expansion and prevent atelectasis through deep breathing and coughing exercises. Frequent meals and supine position may worsen the pain, and morphine is avoided due to its effect on the sphincter of Oddi.

25. Q: Which intervention is a priority for a client in the first hour following a burn injury?

    a) Applying topical antibiotic ointment

    b) Administering intravenous pain medication

    c) Establishing intravenous access for fluid replacement

    d) Administering tetanus prophylaxis

    Answer: c) Establishing intravenous access for fluid replacement

    Explanation: Early fluid replacement is crucial in burn injuries to prevent hypovolemic shock. It is more immediate than pain management and infection prevention at the early stage of burn injury.

26. Q: The nurse is planning care for a client with delirium due to a urinary tract infection. Which intervention is the priority?

    a) Orient the client frequently to time, place, and person.

    b) Encourage family to bring in familiar items from home.

    c) Administer antipsychotic medication as ordered.

    d) Administer antibiotic medication as ordered.

    Answer: d) Administer antibiotic medication as ordered.

    Explanation: The priority for a client with delirium due to UTI is to treat the underlying infection causing the delirium, which is done by administering the prescribed antibiotic medication.

27. Q: Which assessment is a priority for a client receiving heparin therapy?

    a) Blood pressure

    b) Respiratory rate

    c) Activated partial thromboplastin time (aPTT)

    d) Serum potassium level

    Answer: c) Activated partial thromboplastin time (aPTT)

Explanation: aPTT is crucial in monitoring the effectiveness and safety of heparin therapy, helping to adjust the dose to prevent excessive bleeding or inadequate anticoagulation.

28. Q: Which nursing action is most appropriate for a client experiencing an anaphylactic reaction?

    a) Administer antihistamine medication as ordered.

    b) Administer epinephrine as ordered.

    c) Place the client in a high Fowler's position.

    d) Start an IV with a large-bore needle.

    Answer: b) Administer epinephrine as ordered.

Explanation: In an anaphylactic reaction, the priority is to administer epinephrine promptly to reverse life-threatening symptoms like airway swelling and severe hypotension.

29. Q: The nurse is caring for a client with chronic obstructive pulmonary disease (COPD). Which is an appropriate goal?

    a) The client will have a respiratory rate of 30 breaths/min or less.

    b) The client will have oxygen saturation levels above 95%.

    c) The client will be free of dyspnea at rest.

    d) The client will have clear lung sounds in all lobes.

    c) The client will be free of dyspnea at rest.

Explanation: The most appropriate goal for a client with chronic obstructive pulmonary disease (COPD) is to be free of dyspnea at rest. COPD patients often struggle with shortness of breath, and achieving a state where they are not experiencing breathlessness while at rest can significantly improve their quality of life. The other options might not be achievable due to the chronic nature of COPD. The normal respiratory rate and oxygen saturation levels can vary, and clear lung sounds might not be achievable due to chronic changes in the lung tissues associated with COPD.

30. Q: What would be a priority nursing intervention for a patient at risk of deep vein thrombosis?

    a) Encourage mobility

    b) Apply warm compresses

    c) Administer anti-inflammatory medication

    d) Elevate the legs

    Answer: a) Encourage mobility

    Explanation: Elevating the legs can aid in increasing venous return to the heart, which is critical in maintaining blood pressure and cardiac output in a patient in shock.

31. Q: Which of the following is the most appropriate intervention for a patient exhibiting signs of shock?

    a) Elevate the legs

    b) Administer a diuretic

    c) Encourage deep breathing exercises

    d) Provide a warm blanket

    Answer: a) Elevate the legs

    Explanation: Performing a 12-lead ECG is pivotal in quickly identifying any signs of myocardial infarction, allowing for immediate intervention and management.

32. Q: Which of the following interventions is crucial for a patient suspected of having a myocardial infarction?

    a) Administer morphine

    b) Perform a 12-lead ECG

    c) Initiate IV access

d) Administer aspirin

Answer: b) Perform a 12-lead ECG

33. Q: A patient is diagnosed with congestive heart failure (CHF). What dietary advice should be given to this patient?

a) High potassium, low sodium

b) High protein, low fat

c) High carbohydrate, low protein

d) High fat, low carbohydrate

Answer: a) High potassium, low sodium

Explanation: Patients with congestive heart failure (CHF) are usually advised to consume a diet high in potassium and low in sodium to manage fluid balance and prevent further complications related to hypertension and edema.

34. Q: A client with a history of seizures is prescribed phenytoin. Which lab value should the nurse monitor closely?

a) Sodium level

b) Potassium level

c) Blood glucose level

d) Serum phenytoin level

Answer: d) Serum phenytoin level

Explanation: Monitoring serum phenytoin level is essential to ensure the drug is at a therapeutic level to control seizures without causing toxicity.

35. Q: The nurse is caring for a patient who has been vomiting for two days. Which of the following is a priority assessment?

a) Skin turgor

b) Bowel sounds

c) Pupil reaction

d) Reflexes

Answer: a) Skin turgor

Explanation: Assessing skin turgor is a priority in a patient who has been vomiting as it helps in determining the level of dehydration.

36. Q: A patient with end-stage renal disease is most at risk for developing which electrolyte imbalance?

a) Hypocalcemia

b) Hyponatremia

c) Hyperkalemia

d) Hypokalemia

Answer: c) Hyperkalemia

Explanation: Patients with end-stage renal disease are at risk for hyperkalemia due to the kidneys' decreased ability to excrete potassium.

37. Q: What is the priority intervention for a patient diagnosed with a flail chest?

a) Administer pain medication

b) Administer oxygen therapy

c) Apply a chest binder

d) Insert a chest tube

Answer: b) Administer oxygen therapy

Explanation: In a patient with flail chest, administering oxygen therapy is a priority to ensure adequate oxygenation as the flail segment can impair ventilation.

38. Q: Which of the following is a common side effect of opioid analgesics?

a) Diarrhea

b) Tachycardia

c) Hypertension

d) Constipation

Answer: d) Constipation

Explanation: Constipation is a common side effect of opioid analgesics due to their effect on reducing bowel motility.

39. Q: Which vaccine is contraindicated in a patient with a severe egg allergy?

a) Hepatitis B

b) Influenza

c) Tetanus

d) Pneumococcal

Answer: b) Influenza

Explanation: The influenza vaccine is traditionally cultured in egg embryos, making it contraindicated for individuals with a severe egg allergy.

40. Q: A patient with a suspected upper GI bleed has a decreased hematocrit. The nurse understands this is due to:

a) Hemodilution

b) Hemolysis

c) Hemoconcentration

d) Hemorrhage

Answer: d) Hemorrhage

Explanation: A decreased hematocrit in the context of a suspected upper GI bleed would typically be attributed to hemorrhage, indicating loss of red blood cells.

41. Q: For a patient with suspected meningitis, what is the priority nursing action?

a) Administering antibiotics

b) Performing a lumbar puncture

c) Isolating the patient

d) Administering antipyretics

Answer: c) Isolating the patient

Explanation: Isolating the patient is a priority to prevent the spread of the infection to others as meningitis can be highly contagious.

42. Q: A nurse is caring for a patient with acute glomerulonephritis. Which of the following dietary selections is most appropriate?

a) High sodium and high protein

b) Low sodium and low protein

c) High potassium and high carbohydrate

d) Low potassium and high fat

Answer: b) Low sodium and low protein

Explanation: A diet low in sodium and protein is usually recommended for patients with acute glomerulonephritis to reduce workload on the kidneys and manage edema.

43. Q: Which of the following is the best indicator of overall kidney function?

a) Blood urea nitrogen (BUN)

b) Serum creatinine

c) Urine specific gravity

d) Serum potassium

Answer: b) Serum creatinine

Explanation: Serum creatinine is considered a more reliable indicator of kidney function as it is not as easily affected by diet, hydration, or tissue breakdown compared to Blood Urea Nitrogen (BUN).

44. Q: A patient with rheumatoid arthritis (RA) complains of joint pain. Which type of medication will likely be ordered to address this complaint?

a) Antibiotic

b) Diuretic

c) Nonsteroidal anti-inflammatory drug (NSAID)

d) Antipyretic

Answer: c) Nonsteroidal anti-inflammatory drug (NSAID)

Explanation: NSAIDs are often used to manage pain and inflammation associated with rheumatoid arthritis due to their anti-inflammatory properties.

45. Q: What is a potential complication of a fracture that requires immediate medical intervention?

a) Compartment syndrome

b) Infection

c) Delayed union

d) Avascular necrosis

Answer: a) Compartment syndrome

Explanation: Compartment syndrome is a medical emergency that requires immediate intervention to prevent irreversible damage to muscles and nerves due to increased pressure within the muscle compartment.

46. Q: Which type of precautions should be implemented for a patient with a Clostridium difficile infection?

a) Droplet precautions

b) Airborne precautions

c) Contact precautions

d) Standard precautions

Answer: c) Contact precautions

Explanation: Contact precautions are required for Clostridium difficile due to the ability of the spores to survive on surfaces and the potential for transmission via contact.

47. Q: For a client with hypothyroidism, which dietary choice is most appropriate?

a) High fiber and low calorie

b) High carbohydrate and high protein

c) Low fiber and high calorie

d) Low protein and high fat

Answer: a) High fiber and low calorie

Explanation: A high fiber and low calorie diet is appropriate for clients with hypothyroidism to manage weight and prevent constipation, which can be a complication of hypothyroidism.

48. Q: When providing tracheostomy care, which action is most important?

a) Suctioning the tracheostomy before cleaning

b) Cleaning the stoma site with hydrogen peroxide

c) Replacing the tracheostomy tube if it becomes dislodged

d) Keeping a spare tracheostomy tube at the bedside

Answer: d) Keeping a spare tracheostomy tube at the bedside

Explanation: Having a spare tracheostomy tube at the bedside is crucial in case the existing tube becomes obstructed or dislodged, ensuring airway patency can be quickly re-established.

49. Q: The nurse is teaching a patient with diabetes mellitus about foot care. Which statement by the patient indicates a need for further teaching?

   a) "I will inspect my feet daily for any cuts or blisters."

   b) "I will wear cotton socks and well-fitting shoes."

   c) "I can use a heating pad on my feet to increase circulation."

   d) "I will not walk barefoot, even indoors."

   Answer: c) " I can use a heating pad on my feet to increase circulation."

Explanation: People with diabetes often have decreased sensitivity in their extremities, especially the feet, due to peripheral neuropathy. Using a heating pad can lead to burns because they may not feel the heat intensity. Therefore, the statement about using a heating pad indicates a need for further teaching regarding safe practices for foot care in diabetes mellitus.

50. Q: What intervention is essential for a patient at risk of aspiration?

   a) Elevate head of the bed to 45 degrees

   b) Encourage coughing and deep breathing

   c) Administer oxygen therapy

   d) Encourage fluid intake

   Answer: a) Elevate head of the bed to 45 degrees

Explanation: Elevating the head of the bed to at least 30 degrees (45 degrees if possible) is crucial for patients at risk of aspiration. This position helps to prevent aspiration of oral secretions or gastric contents into the lungs by utilizing gravity to keep contents down. In contrast, the other options do not directly prevent the risk of material from being aspirated into the lungs

51. Q: Which of the following lab values would indicate impaired liver function?

a) Decreased albumin

b) Increased sodium

c) Decreased potassium

d) Increased calcium

Answer: a) Decreased albumin

Explanation: Decreased albumin is indicative of impaired liver function because albumin is a protein that is synthesized by the liver. When the liver is impaired, it can't produce albumin effectively, leading to decreased levels in the blood. The other options are not direct indicators of liver function, as they are primarily related to kidney function and electrolyte balance.

52. Q: A nurse is educating a patient with gastroesophageal reflux disease (GERD). Which dietary choice should the patient avoid?

a) Grilled chicken

b) Spaghetti with tomato sauce

c) Baked potato

d) Steamed vegetables

Answer: b) Spaghetti with tomato sauce

Explanation: Patients with gastroesophageal reflux disease (GERD) should avoid foods that can trigger or worsen their symptoms. These typically include acidic, spicy, and fatty foods.

- **Spaghetti with Tomato Sauce:** This option is acidic due to the tomato sauce, and acidic foods can trigger GERD symptoms by increasing stomach acid production, making this a poor choice for someone with GERD.

The other options, like grilled chicken, baked potatoes, and steamed vegetables, are considered more neutral and less likely to provoke GERD symptoms, making them safer dietary choices for individuals with this condition.

53. Q: What intervention is vital for a patient diagnosed with a detached retina?

a) Administer eye drops

b) Place in a prone position

c) Apply a warm compress

d) Maintain strict bed rest

Answer: d) Maintain strict bed rest

Explanation: For patients with a detached retina, maintaining strict bed rest is crucial to prevent further movement and agitation that could worsen the detachment.

54. Q: Which clinical manifestation is a late sign of increased intracranial pressure (ICP)?

a) Nausea

b) Decreased level of consciousness

c) Headache

d) Pupillary asymmetry

Answer: b) Decreased level of consciousness

Explanation: A decreased level of consciousness is a late sign of increased intracranial pressure and is considered a neurological emergency. Early signs might include headache, nausea, and pupillary changes.

55. Q: Which of the following drugs should be avoided in a patient with a history of asthma?

   a) Acetaminophen

   b) Aspirin

   c) Loratadine

   d) Dextromethorphan

   Answer: b) Aspirin

   Explanation: Some asthmatic patients can have aspirin-sensitive asthma, where taking aspirin can trigger asthma symptoms or exacerbate existing symptoms. The other medications listed are generally considered safe for asthmatic individuals.

56. Q: A nurse is monitoring a patient following a thyroidectomy. What complication requires immediate intervention?

   a) Stridor

   b) Hypocalcemia

   c) Hoarseness

   d) Neck swelling

   Answer: a) Stridor

   Explanation: Stridor is a high-pitched, wheezing sound caused by disrupted airflow. It can be indicative of airway obstruction and requires immediate intervention as it can lead to respiratory distress or failure.

57. Q: A patient with pneumonia is receiving antibiotic therapy. What is the best indicator that the treatment is effective?

   a) Normalized white blood cell count

   b) Clear lung sounds

   c) Decreased respiratory rate

   d) Normalized body temperature

Answer: b) Clear lung sounds

Explanation: Clear lung sounds can be a direct indicator that pneumonia is resolving, as pneumonia often causes crackles and other abnormal lung sounds due to the presence of inflammatory exudate. The other options are also important indicators, but clear lung sounds can provide direct evidence of improving lung function and resolving infection.

58. Q: For a client with congestive heart failure, which assessment finding would indicate worsening condition?

a) Decreased peripheral edema

b) Increased urine output

c) Weight gain

d) Decreased respiratory rate

Answer: c) Weight gain

Explanation: Weight gain would indicate a worsening condition as it often signifies fluid retention due to the heart's diminished ability to pump blood efficiently.

59. Q: What is a primary nursing consideration when caring for a patient receiving a blood transfusion?

a) Monitoring for hypotension

b) Administering with dextrose solution

c) Monitoring for a transfusion reaction

d) Administering a diuretic post-transfusion

Answer: c) Monitoring for a transfusion reaction

Explanation: Monitoring for a transfusion reaction is a primary nursing consideration because reactions can be life-threatening. A transfusion reaction occurs when the body has an adverse response to blood received. This can cause symptoms like fever, chills, rash, or breathing difficulties. Immediate detection and intervention are crucial to prevent severe complications, making it essential for nurses to closely monitor patients for any signs of a reaction during a blood transfusion.

60. Q: Which of the following findings is typical for a patient with Cushing's syndrome?

   a) Hypotension

   b) Hypoglycemia

   c) Truncal obesity

   d) Muscle wasting

Answer: c) Truncal obesity

Explanation: Cushing's syndrome is characterized by an excess of cortisol, leading to symptoms like truncal obesity, where there is a disproportionate amount of fat stored in the trunk of the body.

61. Q: What is the most important nursing intervention for a patient with Myasthenia Gravis experiencing a myasthenic crisis?

   a) Administering cholinesterase inhibitors

   b) Initiating mechanical ventilation

   c) Administering immunosuppressive agents

   d) Monitoring vital capacity

Answer: b) Initiating mechanical ventilation

Explanation: In a myasthenic crisis, a severe exacerbation of muscle weakness occurs, affecting the respiratory muscles and leading to respiratory failure. Initiating mechanical ventilation is crucial to maintain adequate ventilation and oxygenation.

62. Q: For a patient with a history of chronic obstructive pulmonary

disease (COPD), which of the following would indicate acute respiratory distress?

a) Decreased respiratory rate

b) Decreased use of accessory muscles

c) Increased oxygen saturation

d) Pursed-lip breathing

Answer: d) Pursed-lip breathing

Explanation: Pursed-lip breathing is a technique used by COPD patients to improve ventilation and reduce dyspnea, and it can indicate that a patient is experiencing increased respiratory distress.

63. Q: A patient is experiencing an acute asthma attack. What medication should the nurse prepare to administer?

a) Albuterol

b) Montelukast

c) Fluticasone

d) Salmeterol

Answer: a) Albuterol

- **Explanation:** Albuterol is a short-acting beta-agonist that can provide quick relief by relaxing the muscles around the airways, making it a first-line medication for acute asthma attacks.

64. Q: A patient is admitted with suspected meningitis. Which of the following is a priority nursing intervention?

a) Administer antibiotics immediately

b) Obtain blood cultures

c) Perform a neurologic assessment

d) Administer antipyretics

Answer: b) Obtain blood cultures

Explanation: While timely administration of antibiotics is crucial in meningitis, obtaining blood cultures before starting antibiotics is essential to identify the causative organism

65. Q: Which medication should be administered to a patient experiencing an anaphylactic reaction?

a) Diphenhydramine

b) Epinephrine

c) Albuterol

d) Hydrocortisone

Answer: b) Epinephrine

Explanation: Epinephrine is the first-line treatment for anaphylaxis as it rapidly alleviates severe allergic reaction symptoms by constricting blood vessels and relaxing smooth muscles in the lungs.

66. Q: For a patient with a spinal cord injury, what is a significant complication to monitor for?

a) Neurogenic shock

b) Increased intracranial pressure

c) Hemorrhagic shock

d) Pulmonary embolism

Answer: a) Neurogenic shock

Explanation: Neurogenic shock is a significant and life-threatening complication of spinal cord injuries, particularly those occurring at or above the T6 level, characterized by hypotension and bradycardia.

67. Q: A nurse is caring for a patient with a new colostomy. What is the priority nursing intervention?

a) Assessing stoma viability

b) Teaching about dietary restrictions

c) Encouraging fluid intake

d) Managing pain

Answer: a) Assessing stoma viability

Explanation: The priority is to assess stoma viability to ensure adequate blood flow to the new stoma, preventing necrosis and other complications.

68. Q: A patient with acute kidney injury (AKI) has a high potassium level. Which medication should the nurse anticipate administering?

a) Furosemide

b) Kayexalate

c) Sodium bicarbonate

d) Calcium gluconate

Answer: b) Kayexalate

Explanation: Kayexalate helps lower high potassium levels by exchanging sodium ions for potassium ions in the intestine and is used in AKI when hyperkalemia is present.

69. Q: What is a major complication associated with abrupt discontinuation of corticosteroid therapy?

a) Hyperglycemia

b) Adrenal crisis

c) Cushing's syndrome

d) Hypertension

Answer: b) Adrenal crisis

Explanation: Abrupt cessation of corticosteroids can lead to adrenal crisis due to the suppressed endogenous cortisol production, a life-threatening condition characterized by hypotension, dehydration, and electrolyte imbalances.

70. Q: A patient with Crohn's disease would benefit most from which type of diet?

   a) High fiber, low fat

   b) High protein, low residue

   c) Low carbohydrate, high fat

   d) High calorie, low protein

   Answer: b) High protein, low residue

   Explanation: A high protein, low residue diet is typically recommended for Crohn's disease patients to provide needed nutrients while reducing intestinal residue and minimizing bowel stimulation.

71. Q: A patient has a burn injury affecting the entire depth of the skin but not underlying tissues. This burn is classified as:

   a) Superficial

   b) Superficial partial-thickness

   c) Deep partial-thickness

   d) Full-thickness

   Answer: c) Deep partial-thickness

   Explanation: Deep partial-thickness burns affect the entire depth of the dermis but spare some underlying structures, causing severe pain, blistering, and a mottled, red to white appearance.

72. Q: Which is a common complication in patients with uncontrolled diabetes mellitus?

   a) Hypoglycemia

   b) Hypotension

   c) Diabetic ketoacidosis

   d) Respiratory alkalosis

   Answer: c) Diabetic ketoacidosis

Explanation: Diabetic ketoacidosis is a severe complication occurring due to a lack of insulin, leading to high blood glucose levels, ketone body accumulation, and metabolic acidosis.

73. Q: For a patient with a deep vein thrombosis (DVT), which medication should be administered as initial treatment?

a) Warfarin

b) Aspirin

c) Heparin

d) Clopidogrel

Answer: c) Heparin

Explanation: Heparin is typically the initial medication of choice for DVT due to its rapid onset of action to prevent further clot formation and growth.

74. Q: A patient with acute pancreatitis should be positioned in which of the following ways to decrease pain?

a) Supine with legs elevated

b) Prone with head elevated

c) Left lateral decubitus

d) Fowler's position

Answer: d) Fowler's position

Explanation: Placing patients with acute pancreatitis in Fowler's position can help reduce pain by decreasing pressure on the abdomen and improving lung expansion.

75. Q: Which of the following is a potential side effect of doxorubicin, an antineoplastic medication?

a) Cardiotoxicity

b) Hypoglycemia

c) Hyperkalemia

d) Constipation

Answer: a) Cardiotoxicity

Explanation: Doxorubicin is known for its potential cardiotoxic side effects, which may include heart failure.

76. Q: A patient with acute glaucoma should avoid which class of medications?

a) Beta-blockers

b) Mydriatics

c) Carbonic anhydrase inhibitors

d) Prostaglandin analogs

Answer: b) Mydriatics

Explanation: Mydriatics dilate the pupils and can increase intraocular pressure, so they are avoided in acute glaucoma.

77. Q: For a patient with a fractured hip, which type of surgical intervention is typically performed?

a) Arthroscopy

b) Hip arthroplasty

c) Lumbar laminectomy

d) Bone grafting

Answer: b) Hip arthroplasty

Explanation: A hip arthroplasty, or hip replacement, is typically performed for patients with fractured hips to restore function and relieve pain.

78. Q: A patient with tuberculosis (TB) should be placed in which type of isolation?

a) Droplet

b) Airborne

c) Contact

d) Protective

Answer: b) Airborne

Explanation: Patients with TB are placed in airborne isolation due to the risk of spreading the infection through tiny droplets expelled into the air.

79. Q: Which assessment finding in a patient with cirrhosis indicates the presence of hepatic encephalopathy?

a) Asterixis

b) Ascites

c) Spider angiomas

d) Palmar erythema

Answer: a) Asterixis

Explanation: Asterixis is a motor disturbance seen in hepatic encephalopathy, associated with cirrhosis, characterized by involuntary flapping of the hands.

80. Q: Which electrolyte imbalance is a common side effect of furosemide?

a) Hypercalcemia

b) Hyperkalemia

c) Hypomagnesemia

d) Hyponatremia

Answer: d) Hyponatremia

Explanation: Furosemide is a loop diuretic that promotes the excretion of sodium and water. Consequently, it can lead to hyponatremia.

81. Q: In which type of shock is the administration of antihistamines most appropriate?

a) Cardiogenic shock

b) Anaphylactic shock

c) Septic shock

d) Hypovolemic shock

Answer: b) Anaphylactic shock

Explanation: Anaphylactic shock is a severe allergic reaction. Antihistamines can help counteract the allergic response.

82. Q: A patient with hyperthyroidism is at risk for which of the following cardiovascular issues?

a) Bradycardia

b) Hypotension

c) Atrial fibrillation

d) Decreased cardiac output

Answer: c) Atrial fibrillation

Explanation: Hyperthyroidism can increase the risk of atrial fibrillation due to its effects on the cardiovascular system.

83. Q: Which intervention is critical for a patient with Guillain-Barré syndrome?

a) Cardiac monitoring

b) Respiratory support

c) Seizure precautions

d) Pain management

Answer: b) Respiratory support

Explanation: Guillain-Barré syndrome can lead to respiratory failure, making respiratory support essential.

84. Q: A patient with multiple sclerosis is experiencing muscle spasticity. Which medication is commonly used to manage this symptom?

a) Baclofen

b) Prednisone

c) Interferon beta-1a

d) Glatiramer acetate

Answer: a) Baclofen

Explanation: Baclofen is a muscle relaxant that can help alleviate muscle spasticity commonly seen in MS patients.

85. Q: Which clinical manifestation is common in patients with rheumatoid arthritis?

a) Hyperuricemia

b) Morning stiffness

c) Subcutaneous nodules

d) Bone spur formation

Answer: b) Morning stiffness

Explanation: Morning stiffness lasting more than 30 minutes is a classic symptom of rheumatoid arthritis.

86. Q: A patient with a brain tumor is exhibiting signs of increased intracranial pressure (ICP). Which medication is administered to decrease ICP?

a) Mannitol

b) Dexamethasone

c) Phenobarbital

d) Morphine

Answer: a) Mannitol

Explanation: Mannitol is an osmotic diuretic that can help reduce ICP.

87. Q: Which is a priority nursing intervention for a patient who has just returned from having a bronchoscopy?

a) Administering prescribed antibiotics

b) Monitoring oxygen saturation levels

c) Encouraging deep breathing exercises

d) Assessing for the return of the gag reflex

Answer: d) Assessing for the return of the gag reflex

Explanation: After bronchoscopy, it's crucial to ensure that the gag reflex has returned before giving anything orally to prevent aspiration.

88. Q: A patient with Addison's disease would primarily benefit from which type of therapy?

a) Insulin therapy

b) Hormone replacement therapy

c) Antihypertensive therapy

d) Diuretic therapy

Answer: b) Hormone replacement therapy

Explanation: Addison's disease is characterized by inadequate adrenal hormone production, requiring hormone replacement therapy.

89. Q: What condition is indicated by a sudden drop in hematocrit in a patient with a burn injury?

a) Hemolysis

b) Hemorrhage

c) Fluid shift

d) Infection

Answer: c) Fluid shift

Explanation: In the early phase after a significant burn, there's a shift of fluid from the intravascular space to the interstitial space, which can cause hemoconcentration and a temporary rise in hematocrit. As fluid is resuscitated, the hematocrit may drop suddenly.

90. Q: Which medication is used as a first-line treatment for a patient with newly diagnosed hypertension?
   a) Atenolol
   b) Clonidine
   c) Hydrochlorothiazide
   d) Nifedipine
   Answer: c) Hydrochlorothiazide
   Explanation: Hydrochlorothiazide is a thiazide diuretic and is commonly used as a first-line treatment for hypertension.

91. Q: Which assessment finding would be expected in a patient with acute pericarditis?
   a) Pulsus paradoxus
   b) Pericardial friction rub
   c) Muffled heart sounds
   d) Widened pulse pressure
   Answer: b) Pericardial friction rub
   Explanation: The sound of pericardial friction rub, caused by the inflamed layers of the pericardium rubbing against each other, is characteristic of acute pericarditis.

92. Q: What is a common complication of long-term opioid use for chronic pain management?
   a) Hyperalgesia
   b) Tolerance

c) Dependence

d) Addiction

Answer: b) Tolerance

Explanation: Tolerance is a common complication of long-term opioid use, requiring increased doses to achieve the same effect.

93. Q: A patient with osteoarthritis is scheduled for a total knee replacement. What is the priority preoperative teaching?

a) Use of assistive devices

b) Pain management

c) Physical therapy exercises

d) Wound care

Answer: c) Physical therapy exercises

Explanation: Learning physical therapy exercises is crucial before surgery to familiarize the patient with postoperative rehabilitation.

94. Q: Which type of isolation is necessary for a patient with Clostridioides difficile (C. diff) infection?

a) Airborne

b) Droplet

c) Contact

d) Protective

Answer: c) Contact

Explanation: Contact isolation is necessary for C. diff infection due to the risk of spreading via contact with spores.

95. Q: What is a characteristic feature of Parkinson's disease?

a) Hyperreflexia

b) Resting tremor

c) Spasticity

d) Rapid eye movement (REM) sleep behavior disorder

Answer: b) Resting tremor

Explanation: Resting tremor is a characteristic feature of Parkinson's disease.

96. Q: Which of the following is a priority intervention for a patient with hypovolemic shock?

a) Administering antibiotics

b) Fluid resuscitation

c) Pain management

d) Administering vasopressors

Answer: b) Fluid resuscitation

Explanation: Fluid resuscitation is the priority intervention in hypovolemic shock to restore intravascular volume.

97. Q: A patient with myasthenia gravis is at risk for which of the following complications?

a) Respiratory failure

b) Renal failure

c) Liver failure

d) Heart failure

Answer: a) Respiratory failure

Explanation: Myasthenia gravis can lead to weakness of the respiratory muscles, causing respiratory failure.

98. Q: Which assessment finding indicates potential hypoxia in a post-operative patient?

a) Bradycardia

b) Hypertension

c) Restlessness

d) Hypothermia

Answer: c) Restlessness

Explanation: Restlessness can be an early sign of hypoxia as the brain is sensitive to changes in oxygen levels.

99. Q: A patient with sepsis has a low blood pressure unresponsive to fluid resuscitation. Which medication is indicated in this scenario?

a) Dobutamine

b) Norepinephrine

c) Amiodarone

d) Furosemide

Answer: b) Norepinephrine

Explanation: Norepinephrine is indicated to increase blood pressure in septic patients unresponsive to fluid resuscitation.

100. Q: A patient with an abdominal aortic aneurysm is at highest risk for which of the following complications?

a) Rupture

b) Thrombosis

c) Embolization

d) Dissection

Answer: a) Rupture

Explanation: Rupture is the most severe complication of an abdominal aortic aneurysm and is a life-threatening emergency.

101. Q: Which of the following interventions is important for a patient diagnosed with congestive heart failure (CHF)?

a) Fluid restriction

b) High-sodium diet

c) Fluid overload

d) High-potassium diet

Answer: a) Fluid restriction

Explanation: Fluid restriction is important in managing congestive heart failure (CHF) to prevent fluid overload and worsening of symptoms.

102. Q: Which type of insulin has the quickest onset of action?

a) Regular insulin

b) NPH insulin

c) Insulin glargine

d) Insulin lispro

Answer: d) Insulin lispro

Explanation: Insulin lispro is a rapid-acting insulin with the quickest onset of action, usually within 15 minutes after injection.

103. Q: What type of fracture is characterized by a bone fragment pulled off by a tendon or ligament?

a) Oblique

b) Avulsion

c) Comminuted

d) Spiral

Answer: b) Avulsion

Explanation: An avulsion fracture is characterized by a piece of bone being pulled away by a tendon or ligament.

104. Q: Which term describes the inability to recognize familiar objects or people?

a) Apraxia

b) Agnosia

c) Anomia

d) Aphasia

Answer: b) Agnosia

Explanation: Agnosia is the inability to recognize familiar objects or people despite intact sensory functions.

105. Q: Which action is most appropriate for a patient diagnosed with Cushing's syndrome?

a) Restricting fluids

b) Administering corticosteroids

c) Monitoring blood glucose levels

d) Administering antithyroid medications

Answer: c) Monitoring blood glucose levels

Explanation: Cushing's syndrome can lead to hyperglycemia; therefore, monitoring blood glucose levels is crucial.

106. Q: Which type of seizure is characterized by a brief loss of consciousness and staring spells?

a) Tonic-clonic

b) Absence

c) Myoclonic

d) Atonic

Answer: b) Absence

Explanation: Absence seizures are characterized by a brief loss of consciousness and staring spells, usually without other motor symptoms.

107. Q: A patient with suspected meningitis exhibits neck rigidity and involuntary hip and knee flexion when the neck is flexed. This sign is known as:

a) Kernig's sign

b) Brudzinski's sign

c) Babinski sign

d) McBurney's sign

Answer: b) Brudzinski's sign

Explanation: Brudzinski's sign is positive when involuntary hip and knee flexion occurs with neck flexion and is indicative of meningeal irritation.

108. Q: For a patient with asthma, which medication is used for quick relief of acute symptoms?

a) Montelukast

b) Albuterol

c) Fluticasone

d) Salmeterol

Answer: b) Albuterol

Explanation: Albuterol is a short-acting beta-agonist used for quick relief of acute asthma symptoms.

109. Q: Which of the following best describes the pain associated with a duodenal ulcer?

a) Sudden, sharp, and severe

b) Burning and cramp-like, relieved by eating

c) Gradual, dull, and achy, aggravated by eating

d) Intermittent, stabbing, and radiating to the back

Answer: b) Burning and cramp-like, relieved by eating

Explanation: Pain from duodenal ulcers is often described as burning and cramp-like and is typically relieved by eating.

110. Q: Which part of the brain is responsible for regulating temperature, hunger, and thirst?

a) Cerebellum

b) Medulla oblongata

c) Hypothalamus

d) Pons

Answer: c) Hypothalamus

Explanation: The hypothalamus is responsible for regulating several physiological functions, including temperature, hunger, and thirst, by maintaining homeostasis.

111. Q: Which of the following conditions is a risk factor for the development of deep vein thrombosis (DVT)?

a) Hyperactivity

b) Dehydration

c) Immobility

d) Hypertension

Answer: c) Immobility

Explanation: Immobility is a significant risk factor for the development of DVT as it can lead to stasis of blood, promoting clot formation.

112. Q: Which intervention is most appropriate for a patient with a pulmonary embolism?

a) Administration of beta-blockers

b) Administration of anticoagulants

c) Encouraging deep breathing exercises

d) Administration of diuretics

Answer: b) Administration of anticoagulants

Explanation: Administering anticoagulants is crucial to prevent further clot formation and propagation in patients with pulmonary embolism.

113. Q: Which diagnostic test is used to confirm a diagnosis of a myocardial infarction (MI)?

a) Electrocardiogram (ECG)

b) Chest X-ray

c) Echocardiogram

d) Cardiac enzyme levels

Answer: d) Cardiac enzyme levels

Explanation: Elevated cardiac enzyme levels, specifically troponins, are confirmatory for myocardial infarction.

114. Q: What is the priority intervention for a patient with acute renal failure?

a) Monitor fluid balance

b) Monitor blood glucose levels

c) Administer anti-hypertensive medications

d) Encourage high-protein diet

Answer: a) Monitor fluid balance

Explanation: Monitoring fluid balance is crucial in managing acute renal failure to avoid fluid overload and to assess kidney function.

115. Q: A patient diagnosed with diverticulitis should avoid consuming which of the following?

a) High-fiber foods

b) Dairy products

c) Seeds and nuts

d) Lean meats

Answer: c) Seeds and nuts

Explanation: Patients with diverticulitis should avoid seeds and nuts, as these can irritate or become trapped in the diverticula.

116. Q: Which clinical manifestation is commonly observed in a patient with hypocalcemia?
  a) Tachycardia
  b) Hyperreflexia
  c) Muscle weakness
  d) Constipation
  Answer: b) Hyperreflexia

117. Q: Which of the following medications is a common treatment for a patient with bipolar disorder?
  a) Lithium
  b) Sertraline
  c) Risperidone
  d) Methylphenidate
  Answer: a) Lithium

118. Q: What is a typical feature of a tension headache?
  a) Pulsating pain on one side of the head
  b) Band-like pain around the head
  c) Sharp, stabbing pain in the eye area
  d) Throbbing pain at the base of the skull
  Answer: b) Band-like pain around the head

119. Q: Which of the following is a common complication associated with a radical mastectomy?
  a) Hemorrhage
  b) Lymphedema

c) Pulmonary embolism

d) Infection

Answer: b) Lymphedema

120. Q: Which intervention is a priority for a patient experiencing alcohol withdrawal?

a) Administering benzodiazepines

b) Encouraging participation in group therapy

c) Administering antipsychotic medications

d) Restricting fluids to avoid fluid overload

Answer: a) Administering benzodiazepines

Explanation: Benzodiazepines are the first-line treatment for managing withdrawal symptoms in patients experiencing alcohol withdrawal

121. Q: Which action is crucial when caring for a patient with a suspected stroke?

a) Performing a thorough neurological assessment

b) Starting cardiopulmonary resuscitation (CPR)

c) Administering aspirin to prevent clot formation

d) Transporting the patient to a stroke center immediately

Answer: d) Transporting the patient to a stroke center immediately

Explanation: Immediate transport to a stroke center is crucial for a suspected stroke to initiate prompt evaluation and management.

122. Q: Which sign is indicative of a positive Romberg test?

a) Inability to touch the nose with eyes closed

b) Loss of balance when standing with feet together and eyes closed

c) Inability to walk heel-to-toe in a straight line

d) Uncoordinated movements when performing rapid alternating movements

Answer: b) Loss of balance when standing with feet together and eyes closed

Explanation: A positive Romberg test is indicative of a loss of balance when standing with feet together and eyes closed and is suggestive of a proprioception deficit.

123. Q: What type of diet is recommended for a patient with acute pancreatitis?

a) High-protein diet

b) Low-fat diet

c) High-carbohydrate diet

d) NPO (nothing by mouth)

Answer: d) NPO (nothing by mouth)

Explanation: Patients with acute pancreatitis are typically kept NPO to rest the pancreas and prevent the secretion of pancreatic enzymes.

124. Q: What is the primary purpose of administering a beta-blocker to a patient with heart failure?

a) To increase heart rate

b) To decrease blood pressure

c) To improve cardiac output

d) To decrease myocardial oxygen consumption

Answer: d) To decrease myocardial oxygen consumption

Explanation: Beta-blockers help in reducing myocardial oxygen demand by decreasing heart rate and blood pressure, thereby beneficial in heart failure management.

125. Q: Which of the following is a risk factor for osteoporosis?

a) High calcium intake

b) Regular weight-bearing exercise

c) Postmenopausal status

d) High vitamin D levels

Answer: c) Postmenopausal status

Explanation: Postmenopausal status is a significant risk factor for osteoporosis due to the decline in estrogen levels, affecting bone density.

126. Q: Which action is most appropriate when performing a sterile dressing change?

a) Wearing clean gloves to remove the old dressing

b) Touching only the edges of the sterile field

c) Using the same sterile gloves to apply the new dressing

d) Cleaning the wound from the center outward in a circular motion

Answer: b) Touching only the edges of the sterile field

Explanation: Touching only the edges of the sterile field helps in maintaining the sterility of the field during a dressing change.

127. Q: What condition is characterized by a decrease in all types of blood cells, including red blood cells, white blood cells, and platelets?

a) Leukemia

b) Pancytopenia

c) Thrombocytopenia

d) Anemia

Answer: b) Pancytopenia

Explanation: Pancytopenia is characterized by a reduction in all three blood cell lines: red blood cells, white blood cells, and platelets.

128. Q: Which of the following is a primary concern related to a patient with burn injuries?

a) Infection

b) Hypothermia

c) Hypertension

d) Hyperkalemia

Answer: a) Infection

Explanation: Infection is a primary concern in burn injuries due to the loss of skin integrity, exposing the underlying tissues to microbes.

129. Q: Which of the following respiratory disorders is characterized by irreversible enlargement of the air spaces distal to the terminal bronchioles?

a) Asthma

b) Chronic bronchitis

c) Emphysema

d) Pulmonary fibrosis

Answer: c) Emphysema

Explanation: Emphysema is characterized by the irreversible enlargement of air spaces distal to the terminal bronchioles, leading to reduced elastic recoil.

130. Q: Which of the following conditions is associated with chronic alcohol abuse?

a) Hypoglycemia

b) Hyperkalemia

c) Cirrhosis

d) Hypocalcemia

Answer: c) Cirrhosis

Explanation: Chronic alcohol abuse is a leading cause of cirrhosis, characterized by the replacement of normal liver tissue with scar tissue.

131. Q: What medication is used to treat anaphylactic reactions?
a) Diphenhydramine
b) Albuterol
c) Epinephrine
d) Hydrocortisone
Answer: c) Epinephrine
Explanation: Epinephrine is pivotal for treating anaphylactic reactions, swiftly constraining blood vessels and opening airways.

132. Q: Which of the following is a common manifestation of right-sided heart failure?
a) Pulmonary edema
b) Peripheral edema
c) Paroxysmal nocturnal dyspnea
d) Orthopnea
Answer: b) Peripheral edema
Explanation: Peripheral edema is a hallmark of right-sided heart failure, manifesting due to the accumulation of fluid in extremities from blood backlog.

133. Q: Which intervention is appropriate for a patient diagnosed with benign prostatic hyperplasia (BPH)?
a) Restricting fluid intake
b) Administering alpha-blockers
c) Performing regular prostate massage
d) Administering anti-inflammatory medications
Answer: b) Administering alpha-blockers

Explanation: Alpha-blockers are employed in BPH treatment to ease symptoms by facilitating the relaxation of bladder and prostate muscles.

134. Q: Which electrolyte imbalance is a potential side effect of loop diuretics?

a) Hypercalcemia

b) Hyperkalemia

c) Hypokalemia

d) Hypernatremia

Answer: c) Hypokalemia

Explanation: Loop diuretics induce increased potassium excretion in urine, leading to hypokalemia.

135. Q: Which sign is characteristic of hyperthyroidism?

a) Weight gain

b) Bradycardia

c) Heat intolerance

d) Constipation

Answer: c) Heat intolerance

Explanation: Increased metabolic rate in hyperthyroidism results in heat intolerance

136. Q: Which intervention is a priority for a patient in the acute phase of a sickle cell crisis?

a) Administering iron supplements

b) Encouraging ambulation

c) Providing adequate hydration

d) Administering vitamin B12 injections

Answer: c) Providing adequate hydration

Explanation: Adequate hydration is crucial during a sickle cell crisis to avoid further sickling of cells.

137. Q: Which clinical manifestation is a classic sign of diabetic ketoacidosis (DKA)?

a) Hypoventilation

b) Hypoglycemia

c) Kussmaul respirations

d) Bradycardia

Answer: c) Kussmaul respirations

Explanation: Kussmaul respirations, characterized by deep and labored breathing, are indicative of DKA.

138. Q: What is a common complication associated with mechanical ventilation?

a) Pneumothorax

b) Pulmonary edema

c) Pleural effusion

d) Pulmonary embolism

Answer: a) Pneumothorax

Explanation: Mechanical ventilation can lead to pneumothorax due to high pressure.

139. Q: Which dietary intervention is important for a patient with gout?

a) Increasing intake of purine-rich foods

b) Increasing protein intake

c) Avoiding alcohol consumption

d) Increasing carbohydrate intake

Answer: c) Avoiding alcohol consumption

Explanation: Alcohol avoidance is advised in gout as it can elevate uric acid levels.

140. Q: Which nursing intervention is essential for a patient receiving enteral nutrition?

a) Administering medications via the feeding tube without flushing

b) Elevating the head of the bed at least 30 degrees during feeding

c) Mixing medications with enteral formula for ease of administration

d) Checking gastric residual volume every 8 hours

Answer: b) Elevating the head of the bed at least 30 degrees during feeding

Explanation: This prevents aspiration during enteral feeding.

141. Q: Which of the following laboratory values is a common finding in a patient with anorexia nervosa?

a) Elevated white blood cell count

b) Elevated blood urea nitrogen (BUN)

c) Low serum potassium

d) Elevated serum glucose

Answer: c) Low serum potassium

Explanation: Anorexia nervosa often results in nutritional deficiencies leading to low serum potassium.

142. Q: Which action is important for reducing the risk of catheter-associated urinary tract infections?

a) Keeping the drainage bag elevated above the level of the bladder

b) Irrigating the catheter daily with an antiseptic solution

c) Emptying the drainage bag at least once per shift

d) Securing the catheter to the thigh with tape

Answer: c) Emptying the drainage bag at least once per shift

Explanation: Regular emptying of the drainage bag helps in preventing urinary tract infections.

143. Q: Which condition is characterized by difficulty in swallowing?

a) Dyspepsia

b) Dysphasia

c) Dysphagia

d) Dyspnea

Answer: c) Dysphagia

Explanation: Dysphagia denotes difficulty in swallowing.

144. Q: Which type of medication is commonly used to treat patients with generalized anxiety disorder (GAD)?

a) Antipsychotic medications

b) Antidepressant medications

c) Antipyretic medications

d) Antispasmodic medications

Answer: b) Antidepressant medications

Explanation: Antidepressants are typically used to manage generalized anxiety disorder.

145. Q: What is the recommended treatment for a patient with acute decompensated heart failure exhibiting pulmonary edema?

a) Administering oral beta-blockers

b) Administering IV diuretics

c) Initiating chest physiotherapy

d) Administering subcutaneous insulin

Answer: b) Administering IV diuretics

Explanation: For acute decompensated heart failure with pulmonary edema, IV diuretics are essential for fluid removal.

146. Q: Which of the following is an early sign of increased intracranial pressure?

a) Hypertension

b) Bradycardia

c) Altered level of consciousness

d) Unequal pupil size

Answer: c) Altered level of consciousness

Explanation: An altered level of consciousness is an early sign of increased intracranial pressure.

147. Q: Which clinical manifestation is indicative of left-sided heart failure?

a) Jugular vein distention

b) Ascites

c) Pulmonary congestion

d) Hepatomegaly

Answer: c) Pulmonary congestion

Explanation: Left-sided heart failure often leads to pulmonary congestion due to blood accumulation in the lungs.

148. Q: Which intervention is recommended for a patient with venous insufficiency?

a) Applying heat to the affected extremity

b) Elevating the legs above the level of the heart

c) Encouraging prolonged sitting or standing

d) Administering anticoagulant medication

Answer: b) Elevating the legs above the level of the heart

Explanation: This assists in reducing edema associated with venous insufficiency.

149. Q: Which medication is used to treat Parkinson's disease by increasing the level of dopamine in the brain?

a) Baclofen

b) Levodopa

c) Gabapentin

d) Phenobarbital

Answer: b) Levodopa

Explanation: Levodopa is utilized in Parkinson's treatment to augment dopamine levels in the brain.

150. Q: What is the priority intervention for a patient who has ingested a corrosive poison?

a) Inducing vomiting

b) Administering activated charcoal

c) Diluting with milk or water

d) Administering a laxative

Answer: c) Diluting with milk or water

Explanation: Dilution is critical for corrosive poison ingestion to mitigate corrosive damage.

151. Q: What intervention is critical for a patient diagnosed with Myasthenia Gravis during a myasthenic crisis?

a) Administering Cholinergic drugs

b) Administering Anticholinergic drugs

c) Encouraging physical exercise

d) Restricting fluid intake

Answer: a) Administering Cholinergic drugs

Explanation: Cholinergic drugs are vital during a myasthenic crisis in patients with Myasthenia Gravis to improve muscle strength.

152. Q: What is a priority nursing intervention for a patient with a suspected pulmonary embolism?

    a) Administering anticoagulants

    b) Encouraging coughing and deep breathing

    c) Administering bronchodilators

    d) Positioning the patient flat in bed

    Answer: a) Administering anticoagulants

Explanation: Anticoagulants are crucial for a suspected pulmonary embolism to prevent clot progression.

153. Q: Which symptom is most indicative of hypoglycemia?

    a) Polyuria

    b) Diaphoresis

    c) Polydipsia

    d) Polyphagia

    Answer: b) Diaphoresis

Explanation: Diaphoresis is a typical indicator of hypoglycemia.

154. Q: Which assessment is most important for a patient diagnosed with glaucoma?

    a) Hearing assessment

    b) Visual field assessment

    c) Taste assessment

    d) Smell assessment

    Answer: b) Visual field assessment

Explanation: This is crucial in glaucoma patients to assess the extent of peripheral vision loss.

155. Q: What intervention is most important for preventing pressure ulcers in immobilized patients?

   a) Keeping the patient dry and clean

   b) Applying topical antibiotics to red areas

   c) Massaging bony prominences

   d) Using doughnut-type cushions

   Answer: a) Keeping the patient dry and clean

   Explanation: Maintaining cleanliness and dryness is fundamental in preventing pressure ulcers in immobilized patients.

156. Q: Which assessment finding would be of most concern for a patient with a history of chronic obstructive pulmonary disease (COPD)?

   a) Barrel chest

   b) Clubbed fingers

   c) Pursed-lip breathing

   d) Altered level of consciousness

   Answer: d) Altered level of consciousness

   Explanation: In COPD patients, an altered level of consciousness can indicate severe hypoxia and is of significant concern.

157. Q: Which of the following interventions is essential when caring for a patient with renal calculi?

   a) Encouraging fluid restriction

   b) Administering calcium supplements

   c) Encouraging high-calcium diet

   d) Straining all urine

   Answer: d) Straining all urine

Explanation: Straining urine is vital for patients with renal calculi to identify passed stones.

158. Q: Which clinical manifestation is most indicative of a tension pneumothorax?

a) Decreased respiratory rate

b) Tracheal deviation to the unaffected side

c) Presence of breath sounds on the affected side

d) Decreased use of accessory muscles

Answer: b) Tracheal deviation to the unaffected side

Explanation: Tracheal deviation to the unaffected side is indicative of a tension pneumothorax.

159. Q: Which of the following is a late sign of hypoxia?

a) Cyanosis

b) Restlessness

c) Tachycardia

d) Hypertension

Answer: a) Cyanosis

Explanation: Cyanosis is a late sign of hypoxia indicating severe oxygen depletion.

160. Q: What clinical manifestation is indicative of right-sided heart failure?

a) Crackles in the lungs

b) Ascites

c) Pulmonary edema

d) Pleural effusion

Answer: b) Ascites

Explanation: Ascites, the accumulation of fluid in the abdominal cavity, is indicative of right-sided heart failure.

161. Q: What is the priority nursing intervention for a patient who has had a cerebrovascular accident (CVA) with right-sided weakness?

a) Initiating seizure precautions

b) Placing the patient in a prone position

c) Performing passive range-of-motion exercises to the right side

d) Maintaining NPO status until a swallow study can be performed

Answer: d) Maintaining NPO status until a swallow study can be performed

Explanation: The priority is to prevent aspiration, and NPO status is maintained until the patient's ability to swallow has been assessed.

162. Q: Which symptom is indicative of the hyperosmolar hyperglycemic state (HHS)?

a) Rapid, deep respirations

b) Decreased urine output

c) Dehydration

d) Fruity breath odor

Answer: c) Dehydration

Explanation: Dehydration is a hallmark of HHS due to excessive urination and fluid loss.

163. Q: What is a major risk factor for developing acute kidney injury?

a) Hypercalcemia

b) Hypotension

c) Hypokalemia

d) Hypoxia

Answer: b) Hypotension

Explanation: Reduced blood flow to the kidneys due to hypotension can lead to acute kidney injury.

164. Q: Which of the following is the most effective measure to prevent the spread of infection?

a) Wearing gloves at all times

b) Hand hygiene

c) Wearing masks

d) Administering antibiotics prophylactically

Answer: b) Hand hygiene

Explanation: Proper hand hygiene is the most effective measure to prevent the spread of infections.

165. Q: What should the nurse include when providing education to a patient with pernicious anemia?

a) Importance of iron supplementation

b) Need for lifelong vitamin B12 injections

c) Benefits of a diet high in folic acid

d) Encouraging intake of vitamin C-rich foods

Answer: b) Need for lifelong vitamin B12 injections

Explanation: Pernicious anemia is caused by a lack of intrinsic factor, leading to vitamin B12 deficiency; thus, lifelong B12 injections are needed.

166. Q: Which intervention is a priority for a patient diagnosed with a hemorrhagic stroke?

a) Administering thrombolytic agents

b) Maintaining a patent airway

c) Encouraging ambulation

d) Monitoring blood glucose levels

Answer: b) Maintaining a patent airway

Explanation: In hemorrhagic stroke, the priority is to maintain a patent airway to ensure adequate oxygenation and ventilation.

167. Q: What clinical manifestation is common in patients with hypothyroidism?

a) Diarrhea

b) Insomnia

c) Weight loss

d) Fatigue

Answer: d) Fatigue

Explanation: Hypothyroidism slows body processes causing fatigue, sluggishness, and tiredness.

168. Q: Which of the following is a common side effect of opioid analgesics?

a) Tachycardia

b) Hypertension

c) Constipation

d) Insomnia

Answer: c) Constipation

Explanation: Opioid analgesics decrease bowel motility leading to constipation.

169. Q: Which electrolyte imbalance is a common complication of diuretic therapy?

a) Hypernatremia

b) Hypercalcemia

c) Hypokalemia

d) Hyperkalemia

Answer: c) Hypokalemia

Explanation: Diuretic therapy can lead to the loss of potassium, resulting in hypokalemia.

170. Q: Which of the following conditions is a contraindication for the administration of a live vaccine?

a) Pregnancy

b) Diabetes mellitus

c) Hypertension

d) Gout

Answer: a) Pregnancy

Explanation: Live vaccines are contraindicated during pregnancy due to the risk to the fetus.

171. Q: What is the initial intervention for a patient experiencing a seizure?

a) Administering antipyretics

b) Positioning the patient on the side

c) Restraining the patient

d) Inserting an oral airway

Answer: b) Positioning the patient on the side

Explanation: Lateral positioning prevents aspiration during a seizure.

172. Q: Which clinical manifestation is a common finding in patients with active tuberculosis?

a) Hemoptysis

b) Weight gain

c) Bradycardia

d) Hypertension

Answer: a) Hemoptysis

Explanation: Hemoptysis or coughing up blood is a common symptom of active tuberculosis.

173. Q: Which of the following interventions is important for managing a patient with delirium?

a) Restraining the patient for safety

b) Keeping the room brightly lit at all times

c) Providing a quiet and calm environment

d) Encouraging the family to stay away from the patient

Answer: c) Providing a quiet and calm environment

Explanation: A quiet and calm environment can reduce agitation in patients with delirium.

174. Q: Which of the following is a typical sign of digoxin toxicity?

a) Tachycardia

b) Hyperkalemia

c) Visual disturbances

d) Hypertension

Answer: c) Visual disturbances

Explanation: Visual disturbances like yellow or green vision are signs of digoxin toxicity.

175. Q: Which of the following laboratory values would indicate a therapeutic level of anticoagulation for a patient receiving warfarin?

a) PT 12 seconds

b) INR 2.5

c) aPTT 28 seconds

d) Platelet count 150,000/mm^3

Answer: b) INR 2.5

Explanation: An INR of 2.5 is within the therapeutic range for anticoagulation with warfarin.

176. Q: What is the priority nursing intervention for a patient with suspected meningitis?

a) Administering antipyretics

b) Performing a lumbar puncture

c) Initiating droplet precautions

d) Monitoring neurological status

Answer: c) Initiating droplet precautions

Explanation: Droplet precautions prevent the spread of diseases, such as meningitis, that are transmitted by respiratory droplets.

177. Q: Which of the following would be the best source of protein for a patient with liver cirrhosis?

a) Cheese

b) Eggs

c) Red meat

d) Vegetables

Answer: d) Vegetables

Explanation: Vegetables are a good source of protein for patients with liver cirrhosis who need to limit animal proteins.

178. Q: What is the primary purpose of administering corticosteroids to a patient with Addison's disease?

a) To increase blood glucose levels

b) To replace deficient hormones

c) To suppress the immune system

d) To promote diuresis

Answer: b) To replace deficient hormones

Explanation: Addison's disease is characterized by adrenal insufficiency, and corticosteroids replace deficient hormones.

179. Q: Which of the following is a common clinical manifestation of severe anemia?

a) Hypertension

b) Tachycardia

c) Polycythemia

d) Hypercalcemia

Answer: b) Tachycardia

Explanation: Tachycardia can occur in severe anemia due to the heart pumping more rapidly to deliver adequate oxygen to tissues.

180. Q: What is the most effective way to prevent the transmission of HIV?

a) Regular hand hygiene

b) Use of condoms during sexual activity

c) Receiving vaccinations

d) Avoiding sharing personal items

Answer: b) Use of condoms during sexual activity

Explanation: Using condoms is the most effective way to prevent the sexual transmission of HIV.

181. Q: For a patient with chronic kidney disease, which dietary modification is most important?

a) Low protein

b) Low carbohydrate

c) High fat

d) High fiber

Answer: a) Low protein

Explanation: Patients with chronic kidney disease have impaired kidney function which struggles to filter waste products, particularly the byproducts of protein metabolism. A low-protein diet can reduce the workload on the kidneys, potentially slowing the progression of kidney disease.

182. Q: Which intervention is the most appropriate for managing a patient with agitated behavior?

a) Using restraints

b) Providing a quiet and low-stimulus environment

c) Offering frequent high-calorie snacks

d) Encouraging participation in group activities

Answer: b) Providing a quiet and low-stimulus environment

Explanation: For agitated patients, providing a quiet and low-stimulus environment can help in reducing agitation by minimizing sensory overload. This intervention is focused on creating a calm and safe environment to address the patient's emotional state and behavioral responses.

183. Q: What is the priority nursing intervention for a patient who has just undergone a thyroidectomy and is experiencing tingling around the mouth and muscle twitching?

a) Administering calcium gluconate

b) Administering insulin

c) Monitoring blood pressure

d) Monitoring blood glucose levels

Answer: a) Administering calcium gluconate

Explanation: Tingling around the mouth and muscle twitching after thyroidectomy can be indicative of hypocalcemia. Administering calcium gluconate is crucial to treat acute hypocalcemia, restoring calcium levels, and preventing complications like tetany.

184. Q: Which of the following actions is most important when caring for a patient in the immediate post-operative period after abdominal surgery?

a) Encouraging ambulation

b) Encouraging deep breathing and coughing

c) Encouraging fluid intake

d) Monitoring for signs of infection

Answer: b) Encouraging deep breathing and coughing

Explanation: Post abdominal surgery, encouraging deep breathing and coughing is vital. These exercises help prevent atelectasis and pneumonia by promoting lung expansion and secretion clearance, crucial for post-operative recovery.

185. Q: What is the most significant risk factor for the development of colorectal cancer?

a) High-fiber diet

b) History of peptic ulcer disease

c) Family history of the disease

d) Sedentary lifestyle

Answer: c) Family history of the disease

Explanation: A family history of colorectal cancer significantly increases the risk of developing the disease due to potential shared genetic, environmental, and lifestyle factors.

186. Q: Which of the following would be the most appropriate choice of intravenous fluid for a dehydrated patient?

a) 5% Dextrose in Water

b) Lactated Ringer's solution

c) 0.45% Sodium Chloride

d) 25% Albumin

Answer: b) Lactated Ringer's solution

Explanation: This isotonic fluid replenishes fluid and electrolytes, making it suitable for dehydration.

187. Q: What is the primary goal of palliative care?

a) To cure the underlying disease

b) To provide comfort and support

c) To prolong life at any cost

d) To aggressively treat all symptoms

Answer: b) To provide comfort and support

Explanation: Palliative care focuses on improving the quality of life for patients with serious illnesses, rather than curing the disease.

188. Q: Which of the following is a common manifestation of deep vein thrombosis (DVT)?

a) Warmth and redness at the site

b) Decreased circumference of the affected limb

c) Decreased temperature of the affected limb

d) Pallor of the affected limb

Answer: a) Warmth and redness at the site

Explanation: These are classic signs of inflammation, commonly seen with DVT.

189. Q: Which electrolyte should be closely monitored in a patient receiving digoxin therapy?

a) Sodium

b) Calcium

c) Potassium

d) Magnesium

Answer: c) Potassium

Explanation: Digoxin and potassium levels have an inverse relationship. Low potassium can increase digoxin toxicity.

190. Q: Which intervention is most beneficial in preventing ventilator-associated pneumonia?

a) Frequent oral care

b) Placing the patient in Trendelenburg position

c) Administering prophylactic antibiotics

d) Keeping the patient deeply sedated

Answer: a) Frequent oral care

Explanation: This reduces the growth of pathogenic bacteria in the mouth, which can be aspirated and cause pneumonia.

191. Q: Which assessment finding would be consistent with a diagnosis of left-sided heart failure?

a) Peripheral edema

b) Ascites

c) Crackles in the lungs

d) Jugular vein distention

Answer: c) Crackles in the lungs

Explanation: Left-sided heart failure leads to pulmonary congestion, resulting in crackles on auscultation.

192. Q: Which medication class is considered the first-line treatment for hypertension?

a) Beta-blockers

b) Diuretics

c) Calcium channel blockers

d) Angiotensin-converting enzyme (ACE) inhibitors

Answer: b) Diuretics

Explanation: They are often first-line treatments as they reduce blood pressure by eliminating excess fluid and sodium.

193. Q: Which of the following conditions would require contact precautions?

a) Influenza

b) Tuberculosis

c) Scabies

d) Pneumonia

Answer: c) Scabies

Explanation: It's a skin infestation that requires contact precautions to prevent its spread.

194. Q: Which action is a priority for a patient with a chest tube that has been accidentally removed?

a) Clamping the tube

b) Covering the site with a sterile dressing taped on three sides

c) Administering pain medication

d) Applying a tourniquet above the site

Answer: b) Covering the site with a sterile dressing taped on three sides

Explanation: Prevents air from entering the pleural space, which could cause a pneumothorax.

195. Q: What is the most common cause of burn injuries in older adults?

a) Electrical burns

b) Chemical burns

c) Scalds from hot liquids

d) Flame burns

Answer: c) Scalds from hot liquids

Explanation: Older adults are more susceptible to burns from accidental spills due to decreased reflexes and mobility.

196. Q: What is the initial step in managing a patient with suspected carbon monoxide poisoning?

a) Administering 100% oxygen

b) Initiating IV fluid therapy

c) Administering activated charcoal

d) Performing gastric lavage

Answer: a) Administering 100% oxygen

Explanation: Oxygen displaces carbon monoxide from hemoglobin, facilitating its removal from the body.

197. Q: Which of the following is a key sign of hypovolemic shock?

a) Bradycardia

b) Hypertension

c) Tachypnea

d) Bounding pulse

Answer: c) Tachypnea

Explanation: Rapid breathing can occur in hypovolemic shock due to decreased oxygen delivery to tissues.

198. Q: Which of the following statements is correct regarding the administration of a blood transfusion?

a) The transfusion should be completed within 6 hours

b) Vital signs should be monitored every 30 minutes during the transfusion

c) The transfusion should be started slowly for the first 15 minutes

d) The patient should not receive any other IV fluids during the transfusion

Answer: c) The transfusion should be started slowly for the first 15 minutes

Explanation: To monitor for any adverse reactions.

199. Q: Which of the following is a common symptom of right-sided heart failure?

a) Pulmonary edema

b) Cough producing frothy sputum

c) Jugular vein distention

d) Decreased urine output

Answer: c) Jugular vein distention

Explanation: It's a sign of increased central venous pressure, typical in right-sided heart failure.

200. Q: What is a priority nursing intervention for a patient diagnosed with a pulmonary embolism?

a) Administering anticoagulant medications as ordered

b) Encouraging coughing and deep breathing

c) Administering diuretics as ordered

d) Positioning the patient in the high Fowler's position

Answer: a) Administering anticoagulant medications as ordered

Explanation: Prevents further clot formation in cases of pulmonary embolism.

201. Q: What is the primary nursing intervention for a patient diagnosed with a flail chest?

a) Administration of high-flow oxygen

b) Administration of analgesics

c) Application of a chest binder

d) Administration of intravenous fluids

Answer: a) Administration of high-flow oxygen

Explanation: A flail chest results from trauma, leading to instability in the chest wall and impaired ventilation. Administering high-flow oxygen helps ensure adequate oxygenation.

202. Q: Which nursing intervention is most appropriate for a patient experiencing an acute asthma attack?

a) Administering beta-blockers promptly

b) Initiating chest physiotherapy

c) Administering short-acting beta-agonists

d) Encouraging deep-breathing exercises

Answer: c) Administering short-acting beta-agonists

Explanation: These medications relax smooth muscles in the airways, providing quick relief during an acute asthma attack.

203. Q: Which laboratory value is most indicative of renal function?

a) Serum albumin

b) Serum creatinine

c) Blood urea nitrogen (BUN)

d) Hematocrit

Answer: b) Serum creatinine

Explanation: It is more specific to renal function than BUN or other lab values, and elevations can indicate renal impairment or failure

204. Q: What is the recommended position for a patient after a liver biopsy?

   a) Left lateral position

   b) Right lateral position

   c) Supine position

   d) Prone position

   Answer: b) Right lateral position

   Explanation: After a liver biopsy, this position helps apply pressure to the liver to minimize the risk of hemorrhage.

205. Q: Which of the following is a common side effect of opioid analgesics?

   a) Diarrhea

   b) Tachycardia

   c) Constipation

   d) Hypertension

   Answer: c) Constipation

   Explanation: Opioid analgesics often cause reduced bowel motility, leading to constipation.

206. Q: How should the nurse respond to a patient who is experiencing auditory hallucinations?

   a) Ignore the behavior and continue with care.

   b) Ask the patient what the voices are saying.

   c) Inform the patient that the voices are not real.

   d) Restrain the patient for safety.

Answer: b) Ask the patient what the voices are saying.

Explanation: This approach validates the patient's experience and can provide important information about the content of the hallucinations.

207. Q: Which of the following is the primary treatment for a patient with type 1 diabetes mellitus?

a) Oral hypoglycemic agents

b) Insulin therapy

c) Dietary modification

d) Exercise regimen

Answer: b) Insulin therapy

Explanation: Individuals with type 1 diabetes do not produce insulin, so they require exogenous insulin to regulate blood glucose levels.

208. Q: What intervention is crucial when caring for a patient with Cushing's syndrome?

a) Restricting fluid intake

b) Providing a low-sodium diet

c) Encouraging mobility

d) Administering glucose supplements

Answer: b) Providing a low-sodium diet

Explanation: Patients with Cushing's syndrome have elevated cortisol levels which can lead to fluid retention and hypertension; a low-sodium diet can help manage these symptoms.

209. Q: What is the first-line treatment for a patient in ventricular fibrillation?

a) CPR

b) Defibrillation

c) Administration of amiodarone

d) Cardiac catheterization

Answer: b) Defibrillation

Explanation: It is the first-line treatment for ventricular fibrillation, a life-threatening heart rhythm, to restore normal cardiac activity.

210. Q: What is the most important nursing intervention for a patient with suspected stroke?

a) Administering aspirin immediately

b) Positioning the patient on their side

c) Obtaining a CT scan promptly

d) Monitoring blood pressure every 15 minutes

Answer: c) Obtaining a CT scan promptly

Explanation: A quick CT scan can help determine the type and location of a stroke, guiding appropriate treatment.

211. Q: What is a common cause of upper GI bleeding?

a) Gastric ulcer

b) Crohn's disease

c) Diverticulitis

d) Colorectal cancer

Answer: a) Gastric ulcer

Explanation: It can lead to upper GI bleeding, presenting as hematemesis or melena.

212. Q: What is the primary goal of therapeutic communication with a suicidal patient?

a) Persuading the patient not to attempt suicide

b) Offering solutions to the patient's problems

c) Establishing a trusting and supportive relationship

d) Encouraging the patient to express anger

Answer: c) Establishing a trusting and supportive relationship

Explanation: This is foundational for therapeutic communication, especially with suicidal patients, to create a safe environment for discussing sensitive issues.

213. Q: Which of the following dietary selections would be appropriate for a patient with gout?

a) Liver

b) Anchovies

c) Lentils

d) Spinach

Answer: d) Spinach

Explanation: It is a suitable dietary choice for gout patients as it is low in purines, unlike other options listed which are high in purines.

214. Q: What nursing intervention is most appropriate for a patient experiencing alcohol withdrawal?

a) Providing a quiet, dimly lit environment

b) Encouraging participation in group therapy

c) Administering stimulant medications

d) Restraining the patient to prevent self-harm

Answer: a) Providing a quiet, dimly lit environment

Explanation: This can help in reducing agitation and sensory overstimulation in patients experiencing alcohol withdrawal.

215. Q: Which of the following would be the most appropriate initial intervention for a patient who has ingested a corrosive poison?

a) Inducing vomiting

b) Administering activated charcoal

c) Diluting the poison with milk or water

d) Administering an antidote immediately

Answer: c) Diluting the poison with milk or water

Explanation: For corrosive poisons, dilution can help minimize damage to the mucous membranes, whereas inducing vomiting can cause further damage.

216. Q: What is the primary symptom of a tension pneumothorax?

a) Deviated trachea

b) Decreased respiratory rate

c) Bradycardia

d) Hyperresonance on percussion

Answer: a) Deviated trachea

Explanation: In tension pneumothorax, air pressure builds up in the pleural space, shifting the mediastinum and deviating the trachea.

217. Q: Which assessment finding indicates that a nasogastric (NG) tube is in the correct position?

a) Ability to speak clearly

b) Return of gastric content upon aspiration

c) Absence of abdominal distention

d) Presence of bowel sounds

Answer: b) Return of gastric content upon aspiration

Explanation: Explanation: This finding indicates that the NG tube is correctly placed in the stomach because gastric contents are being aspirated. When you insert an NG tube, you want it to end up in the stomach to achieve the desired outcomes.

218. Q: What is the priority nursing intervention for a patient diagnosed with bulimia nervosa?

a) Monitoring during and after meals

b) Encouraging a high-fiber diet

c) Providing nutritional education

d) Administering antidepressant medications

Answer: a) Monitoring during and after meals

Explanation: Explanation: Monitoring during and after meals is essential for patients with bulimia nervosa to prevent purging behaviors, which can have serious health consequences.

219. Q: Which nursing intervention is most important for a patient receiving peritoneal dialysis?

a) Monitoring blood pressure every 15 minutes

b) Ensuring the dialysate is warmed before infusion

c) Administering insulin as prescribed

d) Encouraging a high-protein diet

Answer: b) Ensuring the dialysate is warmed before infusion

Explanation: Warming the dialysate promotes comfort and optimal exchange of waste, electrolytes, and fluids during peritoneal dialysis.

220. Q: What is a typical clinical manifestation of rheumatoid arthritis?

a) Heberden's nodes

b) Symmetrical joint inflammation

c) Scoliosis

d) Crepitus

Answer: b) Symmetrical joint inflammation

Explanation: It's a characteristic feature of rheumatoid arthritis, distinguishing it from other types of arthritis like osteoarthritis which often affects joints asymmetrically.

221. Q: Which of the following is the appropriate first action for a nurse who discovers fire in a patient's room?

a) Activate the fire alarm

b) Extinguish the fire

c) Evacuate the patient

d) Close the doors and windows

Answer: c) Evacuate the patient

Explanation:

222. Q: What is the most appropriate nursing intervention for a patient with Myasthenia Gravis experiencing a myasthenic crisis?

a) Administering additional anticholinesterase medications

b) Encouraging rest and conserving energy

c) Performing chest physiotherapy

d) Administering intravenous immunoglobulin

Answer: b) Encouraging rest and conserving energy

Explanation: Explanation: During a myasthenic crisis, the patient's muscle weakness worsens. The most appropriate nursing intervention is to encourage the patient to rest and conserve energy to prevent further muscle fatigue.

223. Q: What is the most important nursing intervention for a patient with a chest tube?

a) Clamping the tube regularly to check for air leaks

b) Encouraging deep breathing and coughing

c) Maintaining the drainage system below chest level

d) Stripping the tubing to maintain patency

Answer: c) Maintaining the drainage system below chest level

Explanation: Explanation: The chest drainage system must be kept below the level of the patient's chest to facilitate proper drainage and prevent backflow of fluid or air into the chest cavity. This helps maintain the integrity of the chest tube system.

224. Q: What is the primary symptom of infective endocarditis?

a) Chest pain

b) Dyspnea

c) Fever

d) Palpitations

Answer: c) Fever

Explanation: Explanation: Fever is a common symptom of infective endocarditis. It often presents with other symptoms such as fatigue, malaise, and heart murmurs.

225. Q: Which of the following would be most appropriate for managing a patient with delirium due to a urinary tract infection?

a) Administering antipsychotic medications

b) Applying physical restraints

c) Treating the underlying infection

d) Providing sensory stimulation

Answer: c) Treating the underlying infection

Explanation: Explanation: Delirium can be caused by underlying medical conditions like urinary tract infections. Treating the infection is essential to resolving the delirium. Administering antipsychotic medications or applying physical restraints should not be the first-line approach.

226. Q: Which of the following is the most common cause of dementia in the elderly?

a) Huntington's disease

b) Creutzfeldt-Jakob disease

c) Alzheimer's disease

d) Multiple sclerosis

Answer: c) Alzheimer's disease

Explanation: Explanation: Alzheimer's disease is the most common cause of dementia in the elderly population. It is characterized by progressive cognitive decline and memory impairment.

227. Q: Which of the following foods would be most appropriate for a patient with a history of kidney stones?

a) Spinach

b) Chocolate

c) Nuts

d) Rice

Answer: d) Rice

Explanation: Explanation: Rice is a low-oxalate food, making it a suitable choice for patients with a history of kidney stones. High-oxalate foods like spinach, chocolate, and nuts should be consumed in moderation by such patients to reduce the risk of stone formation.

228. Q: Which of the following is a common side effect of radiation therapy?

a) Alopecia

b) Hypertension

c) Tachycardia

d) Hyperkalemia

Answer: a) Alopecia

Explanation: Explanation: Alopecia, or hair loss, is a common side effect of radiation therapy, especially when the therapy is directed at the head or neck region.

229. Q: What is the priority nursing intervention for a patient experiencing an anaphylactic reaction?

a) Administering an antihistamine

b) Administering epinephrine

c) Starting an IV line

d) Administering a steroid

Answer: b) Administering epinephrine

Explanation: Explanation: Administering epinephrine is the top priority in managing an anaphylactic reaction. Epinephrine helps reverse the severe allergic response and can be life-saving.

230. Q: Which of the following interventions is most important for preventing pressure ulcers in immobilized patients?

a) Applying talcum powder to reduce friction

b) Massaging bony prominences regularly

c) Changing the patient's position every two hours

d) Keeping the head of the bed elevated

Answer: c) Changing the patient's position every two hours

Explanation: Explanation: Regularly changing the patient's position is crucial for preventing pressure ulcers in immobilized patients. This helps relieve pressure on vulnerable areas of the skin and promotes circulation.

231. Q: Which is a correct hand hygiene step when using hand sanitizer?

a) Washing hands with water after applying sanitizer

b) Drying hands with a towel after applying sanitizer

c) Rubbing hands together until the sanitizer is dry

d) Applying a small amount of sanitizer

Answer: c) Rubbing hands together until the sanitizer is dry

Explanation: Explanation: When using hand sanitizer, you should rub your hands together until the sanitizer is completely dry. This ensures that the sanitizer has had enough contact time to effectively kill germs.

232. Q: What is a critical nursing action when caring for a patient with a tracheostomy?

    a) Suctioning the tracheostomy every hour

    b) Changing the tracheostomy ties daily

    c) Keeping a spare tracheostomy tube at the bedside

    d) Providing oral care every 8 hours

    Answer: c) Keeping a spare tracheostomy tube at the bedside

    Explanation: Explanation: Keeping a spare tracheostomy tube at the bedside is essential in case of an emergency or if the current tube becomes dislodged or blocked. This helps ensure the patient's airway remains patent.

233. Q: Which of the following is a key component in managing a patient with reactive hypoglycemia?

    a) Encouraging a diet high in simple carbohydrates

    b) Administering regular insulin as needed

    c) Encouraging frequent, small meals

    d) Administering oral hypoglycemic agents

    Answer: c) Encouraging frequent, small meals

    Explanation: Explanation: Managing reactive hypoglycemia involves encouraging the patient to eat frequent, small meals to help stabilize blood sugar levels and prevent episodes of low blood sugar.

234. Q: What is the appropriate intervention for a patient experiencing a sickle cell crisis?

    a) Administration of iron supplements

    b) High-dose vitamin C administration

c) Hydration and pain management

d) Blood transfusion

Answer: c) Hydration and pain management

Managing a sickle cell crisis involves providing adequate hydration to prevent further sickling of red blood cells and managing pain, which is a hallmark of sickle cell crisis

235. Q: What is a key nursing intervention for a patient diagnosed with Guillain-Barré Syndrome?

a) Encouraging physical therapy and mobility

b) Monitoring respiratory function and providing ventilatory support as needed

c) Administering steroids to reduce inflammation

d) Encouraging a high-protein diet

Answer: b) Monitoring respiratory function and providing ventilatory support as needed

Explanation: Guillain-Barré Syndrome can lead to respiratory muscle weakness. Therefore, monitoring respiratory function and providing ventilatory support, if necessary, are critical nursing interventions.

236. Q: What is the priority nursing intervention for a patient with hyperkalemia?

a) Administering sodium polystyrene sulfonate

b) Encouraging intake of potassium-rich foods

c) Administering IV calcium gluconate

d) Administering a loop diuretic

Answer: a) Administering sodium polystyrene sulfonate

Explanation: Administering sodium polystyrene sulfonate helps lower potassium levels by promoting its excretion through the gastrointestinal tract, which is crucial in managing hyperkalemia.

237. Q: Which of the following is the most accurate method for confirming the placement of a nasogastric tube?

    a) Auscultating for a whooshing sound after injecting air

    b) Observing the tube through the nostril to the stomach

    c) Checking the pH of the aspirate

    d) Observing for respiratory distress

    Answer: c) Checking the pH of the aspirate

Explanation: Checking the pH of the aspirate can confirm that the nasogastric tube is in the stomach, as stomach contents are acidic. This is a more reliable method than other techniques like auscultation.

238. Q: What is the most important factor in wound healing?

    a) Age of the patient

    b) Nutritional status

    c) Presence of infection

    d) Wound size

    Answer: b) Nutritional status

Explanation: Nutritional status is a crucial factor in wound healing because the body requires adequate nutrients to support tissue repair and regeneration.

239. Q: Which medication would be most appropriate for a patient experiencing acute anxiety?

    a) Diazepam

    b) Fluoxetine

    c) Lithium carbonate

    d) Haloperidol

    Answer: a) Diazepam

Explanation: Diazepam is a benzodiazepine that can be used to manage acute anxiety and provide relief to the patient.

240. Q: Which of the following is a common sign of left-sided heart failure?

a) Jugular vein distention

b) Peripheral edema

c) Crackles in the lungs

d) Ascites

Answer: c) Crackles in the lungs

Explanation: Left-sided heart failure can lead to pulmonary congestion, which can manifest as crackles or rales in the lungs due to fluid accumulation.

241. Q: Which of the following is a priority nursing intervention for a patient with a history of falls?

a) Encouraging the use of a walker or cane

b) Placing the bed in the lowest position

c) Encouraging the patient to rise quickly from a sitting position

d) Leaving the bedside commode at a distance to encourage mobility

Answer: b) Placing the bed in the lowest position

Explanation: Placing the bed in the lowest position helps reduce the risk of injury if the patient falls out of bed.

242. Q: What is the most appropriate action for a nurse when a patient refuses medication?

a) Coercing the patient to take the medication

b) Documenting the refusal and notifying the healthcare provider

c) Administering the medication in a different form without informing the patient

d) Discarding the medication without documentation

Answer: b) Documenting the refusal and notifying the healthcare provider

Explanation: When a patient refuses medication, it is essential to document the refusal and notify the healthcare provider for further instructions.

243. Q: Which of the following would be most appropriate to include in the teaching plan for a patient with a new colostomy?

a) Avoiding all fruits and vegetables

b) Performing colostomy irrigations daily

c) Restricting fluid intake

d) Encouraging regular skin care around the stoma

Answer: d) Encouraging regular skin care around the stoma

Explanation: Proper skin care around the stoma is essential to prevent skin irritation and breakdown. It is an important aspect of colostomy care.

244. Q: What should a nurse prioritize when caring for a patient with a seizure disorder who is experiencing a seizure?

a) Inserting an oral airway

b) Holding the patient down to prevent injury

c) Timing the duration of the seizure

d) Protecting the patient's head and maintaining airway patency

Answer: d) Protecting the patient's head and maintaining airway patency

Explanation: During a seizure, protecting the patient's head from injury and ensuring a patent airway are the top priorities.

245. Q: Which of the following is a critical nursing action when administering a blood transfusion?

a) Starting the transfusion slowly and staying with the patient for the first 15 minutes

b) Running the blood transfusion at a fast rate to prevent clotting

c) Administering the blood transfusion with dextrose solution

d) Mixing medications in the blood transfusion bag

Answer: a) Starting the transfusion slowly and staying with the patient for the first 15 minutes

Explanation: Starting a blood transfusion slowly and staying with the patient for the first 15 minutes is crucial to monitor for any adverse reactions, such as transfusion reactions.

246. Q: Which of the following is the best indicator of fluid balance in a patient?

a) Blood pressure

b) Heart rate

c) Daily weight

d) Urine output

Answer: c) Daily weight

Explanation: Daily weight is an excellent indicator of fluid balance in a patient. Sudden weight gain or loss can be indicative of fluid retention or dehydration.

247. Q: Which of the following should a nurse monitor in a patient receiving heparin therapy?

a) Prothrombin time (PT)

b) International normalized ratio (INR)

c) Activated partial thromboplastin time (aPTT)

d) Hemoglobin

Answer: c) Activated partial thromboplastin time (aPTT)

Explanation: Monitoring the activated partial thromboplastin time (aPTT) is essential for patients receiving heparin therapy to ensure the therapeutic range and prevent complications such as bleeding.

248. Q: Which of the following is a priority nursing action for a patient with an altered level of consciousness (ALOC)?

a) Monitoring vital signs every 4 hours

b) Placing the patient in a prone position

c) Maintaining a patent airway

d) Providing oral fluids

Answer: c) Maintaining a patent airway

Explanation: Maintaining a patent airway is the top priority for a patient with an altered level of consciousness. Ensuring that the patient can breathe adequately is essential for their

249. Q: When caring for a patient with glaucoma, what is an important teaching point the nurse should emphasize?

a) Administration of eye drops to reduce intraocular pressure

b) Encouraging regular eye examinations to change prescription glasses

c) Avoiding reading and other activities that strain the eyes

d) Informing the healthcare provider of any color vision changes

Answer: a) Administration of eye drops to reduce intraocular pressure

Explanation: Administering eye drops as prescribed is crucial in managing glaucoma and reducing intraocular pressure to prevent further vision loss.

250. Q: What is the priority nursing intervention for a patient with myasthenia gravis experiencing a myasthenic crisis?

a) Administering cholinesterase inhibitors

b) Administering corticosteroids

c) Initiating mechanical ventilation

d) Administering intravenous immunoglobulin

Answer: c) Initiating mechanical ventilation

Explanation: In a myasthenic crisis, respiratory muscles can become severely weakened, necessitating mechanical ventilation to support the patient's breathing. This is a priority intervention.

251. Q: Which of the following is the most appropriate dietary recommendation for a patient with chronic kidney disease?

a) High-protein diet

b) Low-calcium diet

c) Low-potassium diet

d) High-phosphorus diet

Answer: c) Low-potassium diet

Explanation: Patients with chronic kidney disease often need to restrict potassium intake to prevent hyperkalemia, making a low-potassium diet appropriate.

252. Q: What is a key nursing intervention for a patient post-cardiac catheterization?

a) Encouraging ambulation immediately after the procedure

b) Monitoring the catheter insertion site for bleeding or hematoma formation

c) Allowing the patient to consume food and water immediately after the procedure

d) Positioning the patient with the head of the bed elevated 45 degrees

Answer: b) Monitoring the catheter insertion site for bleeding or hematoma formation

Explanation: After a cardiac catheterization, monitoring the catheter insertion site for any signs of bleeding or hematoma formation is crucial to detect and address any potential complications

253. Q: What is the primary nursing intervention for a patient presenting with symptoms of a stroke?

a) Administering aspirin immediately

b) Performing a glucose check

c) Positioning the patient on their left side

d) Initiating antihypertensive therapy

Answer: b) Performing a glucose check

Explanation: Performing a glucose check is essential to rule out hypoglycemia, which can present with stroke-like symptoms. It is a critical step in the assessment of a stroke patient.

254. Q: What would be a priority nursing intervention for a patient with suspected meningitis?

a) Administering antipyretics

b) Starting antibiotic therapy promptly after cultures are obtained

c) Encouraging fluid intake

d) Placing in a room with a positive pressure environment

Answer: b) Starting antibiotic therapy promptly after cultures are obtained

Explanation: Prompt initiation of antibiotic therapy after obtaining cultures is crucial in suspected cases of bacterial meningitis to prevent further complications.

255. Q: Which vitamin is essential for proper blood clotting?

   a) Vitamin A

   b) Vitamin D

   c) Vitamin K

   d) Vitamin E

   Answer: c) Vitamin K

   Explanation: Vitamin K is essential for proper blood clotting as it plays a key role in the coagulation cascade.

256. Q: For a patient with a suspected pulmonary embolism, what is the priority intervention?

   a) Administering oxygen

   b) Administering anticoagulants

   c) Encouraging ambulation

   d) Providing pain relief

   Answer: a) Administering oxygen

   Explanation: Administering oxygen is a priority in a patient with a suspected pulmonary embolism to ensure adequate oxygenation.

257. Q: What is the most critical intervention for a newborn with a suspected congenital heart defect?

   a) Administering digoxin

   b) Providing supplemental oxygen

   c) Starting prophylactic antibiotics

   d) Immediate surgical intervention

   Answer: b) Providing supplemental oxygen

   Explanation: Providing supplemental oxygen is crucial for a newborn with a suspected congenital heart defect to ensure adequate oxygenation while further evaluation and interventions are planned.

258. Q: What is a priority assessment for patients with chronic obstructive pulmonary disease (COPD)?

a) Pulse oximetry

b) Bowel sounds

c) Peripheral pulses

d) Skin turgor

Answer: a) Pulse oximetry

Explanation: Assessing oxygen saturation using pulse oximetry is a priority in patients with COPD to monitor their oxygen levels and respiratory status.

259. Q: What is the first-line treatment for a patient presenting with diabetic ketoacidosis (DKA)?

a) Insulin therapy

b) Oral hypoglycemic agents

c) Bicarbonate administration

d) Intravenous fluids

Answer: a) Insulin therapy

Explanation: The first-line treatment for DKA is insulin therapy to lower blood glucose levels and correct the metabolic imbalance.

260. Q: What is a priority nursing intervention for a patient with hypovolemic shock?

a) Administration of vasopressors

b) Administration of IV fluids

c) Placement in Trendelenburg position

d) Administration of blood products

Answer: b) Administration of IV fluids

Explanation: The first-line treatment for hypovolemic shock is the rapid administration of intravenous (IV) fluids to restore blood volume.

261. Q: What is the appropriate intervention for a patient with a rectal temperature of 105°F (40.5°C)?

a) Applying warm compresses

b) Administering acetaminophen

c) Encouraging increased fluid intake

d) Providing additional blankets

Answer: b) Administering acetaminophen

Explanation: An extremely high rectal temperature indicates fever, and administering acetaminophen can help lower the fever and provide relief.

262. Q: Which lab value is indicative of impaired kidney function?

a) Elevated serum creatinine

b) Decreased blood urea nitrogen (BUN)

c) Decreased white blood cell count

d) Elevated platelet count

Answer: a) Elevated serum creatinine

Explanation: Elevated serum creatinine levels are indicative of impaired kidney function as the kidneys are not effectively filtering creatinine from the blood.

263. Q: What is the priority nursing action for an unconscious patient?

a) Checking blood glucose levels

b) Performing a neurological exam

c) Establishing an IV line

d) Initiating CPR

Answer: a) Checking blood glucose levels

Explanation: Checking blood glucose levels is essential in an unconscious patient to rule out hypoglycemia, which can cause altered consciousness.

264. Q: When caring for a patient with heart failure, which dietary modification is most appropriate?

a) High-protein diet

b) Low-sodium diet

c) High-carbohydrate diet

d) High-fat diet

Answer: b) Low-sodium diet

Explanation: A low-sodium diet is appropriate for patients with heart failure to reduce fluid retention and manage symptoms related to fluid overload.

265. Q: What is the most important nursing intervention for a patient who has undergone a total laryngectomy?

a) Teaching the patient how to speak using an artificial larynx

b) Managing pain effectively

c) Providing emotional support

d) Monitoring for signs of infection

Answer: a) Teaching the patient how to speak using an artificial larynx

Explanation: Teaching the patient how to speak using an artificial larynx is essential after a total laryngectomy to help them communicate effectively, which is vital for their quality of life.

266. Q: Which medication is used as a first-line treatment for hypertensive crisis?

a) Atenolol

b) Nitroprusside

c) Lisinopril

d) Hydrochlorothiazide

Answer: b) Nitroprusside

Explanation: Nitroprusside is a potent vasodilator and is often used as a first-line treatment for hypertensive crisis to rapidly reduce blood pressure.

267. Q: What is the priority nursing action for a patient in ventricular fibrillation?

a) Administering amiodarone IV push

b) Starting cardiopulmonary resuscitation (CPR)

c) Defibrillation

d) Administering epinephrine IV push

Answer: c) Defibrillation

Explanation: The priority in ventricular fibrillation is defibrillation to restore a normal heart rhythm. CPR may also be initiated as part of the resuscitation process.

268. Q: Which of the following is a critical intervention for a patient with acute respiratory distress syndrome (ARDS)?

a) Administering high-flow oxygen

b) Administering corticosteroids

c) Placing the patient in a prone position

d) Administering diuretics

Answer: a) Administering high-flow oxygen

Explanation: Administering high-flow oxygen is crucial in ARDS to ensure adequate oxygenation, as these patients often have severe respiratory distress.

269. Q: What intervention is crucial for a patient diagnosed with tuberculosis?

a) Administering a live vaccine

b) Placing the patient in airborne isolation

c) Administering broad-spectrum antibiotics

d) Performing a bronchoscopy

Answer: b) Placing the patient in airborne isolation

Explanation: Placing the patient in airborne isolation is essential to prevent the spread of tuberculosis, which is transmitted through respiratory droplets.

270. Q: For a patient with severe anemia, what is the priority nursing intervention?

a) Monitoring for signs of infection

b) Administering iron supplements

c) Encouraging increased fluid intake

d) Administering a blood transfusion

Answer: d) Administering a blood transfusion

Explanation: Administering a blood transfusion is the priority for a patient with severe anemia to quickly restore hemoglobin levels and improve oxygen-carrying capacity.

271. Q: Which action is most appropriate for a patient with a pulmonary embolism and hypotension?

a) Administering diuretics

b) Administering anticoagulants

c) Administering vasopressors

d) Encouraging deep-breathing exercises

Answer: c) Administering vasopressors

Explanation: Administering vasopressors is necessary for a patient with a pulmonary embolism and hypotension to increase blood pressure and perfusion to vital organs.

272. Q: When caring for a patient with severe dehydration, what is the priority nursing intervention?

a) Monitoring intake and output

b) Encouraging oral fluid intake

c) Administering IV fluids

d) Monitoring for signs of overhydration

Answer: c) Administering IV fluids

Explanation: Administering IV fluids is the priority for a patient with severe dehydration to rapidly rehydrate and correct electrolyte imbalances.

273. Q: Which intervention is most important for a patient with acute pancreatitis?

a) Administering pain medication

b) Encouraging a low-fat diet

c) Administering insulin

d) Placing the patient in a side-lying position

Answer: a) Administering pain medication

Explanation: Administering pain medication is crucial for a patient with acute pancreatitis to alleviate severe abdominal pain and discomfort.

274. Q: What is the priority nursing action for a patient with an upper gastrointestinal bleed?

a) Starting an IV line

b) Administering a proton pump inhibitor

c) Inserting a nasogastric tube

d) Placing the patient in a semi-Fowler's position

Answer: a) Starting an IV line

Explanation: Starting an IV line is the priority for a patient with an upper gastrointestinal bleed to ensure access for fluids, blood products, and medications as needed.

275. Q: Which of the following interventions is most appropriate for a patient with a deep vein thrombosis (DVT)?

a) Encouraging ambulation

b) Applying warm compresses

c) Administering anticoagulants

d) Performing a massage at the site

Answer: c) Administering anticoagulants

Explanation: Administering anticoagulants is the primary treatment for a patient with a deep vein thrombosis (DVT) to prevent further clot formation and reduce the risk of complications.

276. Q: What is the primary intervention for a patient with acute glomerulonephritis?

a) Administering antibiotics

b) Administering antihypertensive medications

c) Monitoring urine output

d) Encouraging fluid intake

Answer: a) Administering antibiotics

Explanation: Administering antibiotics is the primary intervention for a patient with acute glomerulonephritis, particularly if the cause is bacterial infection.

277. Q: Which of the following interventions is most important for a patient with a head injury?

   a) Monitoring neurological status frequently

   b) Administering pain medication

   c) Encouraging cough and deep breathing exercises

   d) Applying a cold compress to the head

   Answer: a) Monitoring neurological status frequently

Explanation: Monitoring neurological status frequently is critical for a patient with a head injury to assess for changes in level of consciousness or neurological deficits.

278. Q: Which of the following is the priority nursing action for a patient with third-degree burns covering 30% of the body?

   a) Administering intravenous fluids

   b) Applying topical antibiotics

   c) Debriding necrotic tissue

   d) Administering pain medication

   Answer: a) Administering intravenous fluids

Explanation: Administering intravenous fluids is a priority for a patient with extensive burns to maintain circulation and prevent hypovolemic shock.

279. Q: Which of the following interventions is most crucial for a patient with suspected spinal injury?

   a) Administering corticosteroids

   b) Immobilizing the spine

c) Administering muscle relaxants

d) Performing a neurological assessment

Answer: b) Immobilizing the spine

Explanation: Immobilizing the spine is crucial for a patient with suspected spinal injury to prevent further damage to the spinal cord.

280. Q: What is the priority nursing action for a patient experiencing an anaphylactic reaction?

a) Administering an antihistamine

b) Administering epinephrine

c) Administering a steroid

d) Administering a bronchodilator

Answer: b) Administering epinephrine

Explanation: Administering epinephrine is the priority in an anaphylactic reaction to counteract severe allergic reactions and improve cardiovascular and respiratory function.

281. Q: What is the priority nursing intervention for a patient with acute pericarditis?

a) Administering NSAIDs

b) Administering corticosteroids

c) Monitoring cardiac rhythms

d) Placing the patient in Fowler's position

Answer: a) Administering NSAIDs

Explanation: Administering nonsteroidal anti-inflammatory drugs (NSAIDs) is a common intervention for relieving pain and inflammation in acute pericarditis.

282. Q: For a patient with chronic venous insufficiency, which of the following interventions is most appropriate?

a) Applying warm compresses

b) Encouraging leg elevation

c) Administering diuretics

d) Encouraging exercise

Answer: b) Encouraging leg elevation

Explanation: Elevating the legs is a helpful intervention for patients with chronic venous insufficiency to reduce edema and improve venous return.

283. Q: Which medication should be administered immediately to a patient in status epilepticus?

a) Lorazepam (Ativan)

b) Phenobarbital

c) Phenytoin (Dilantin)

d) Valproic acid (Depakote)

Answer: a) Lorazepam (Ativan)

Explanation: Lorazepam (Ativan) is a fast-acting medication used to stop prolonged seizures, such as those in status epilepticus.

284. Q: What is the priority nursing intervention for a patient with a flail chest?

a) Pain management

b) Administration of muscle relaxants

c) Assisted ventilation

d) Application of a chest binder

Answer: c) Assisted ventilation

Explanation: A patient with a flail chest may have impaired breathing due to multiple rib fractures. Assisted ventilation may be necessary to maintain adequate oxygenation and ventilation.

285. Q: What intervention is most crucial for a patient who has ingested a corrosive poison?

a) Administering activated charcoal

b) Inducing vomiting

c) Diluting the poison with milk or water

d) Administering an antidote

Answer: c) Diluting the poison with milk or water

Explanation: Diluting the poison with milk or water is a critical intervention for corrosive poison ingestion to minimize damage to the gastrointestinal tract.

286. Q: Which intervention is most important for a patient diagnosed with Clostridium difficile infection?

a) Encouraging fluid intake

b) Administering probiotics

c) Placing in contact isolation

d) Administering antidiarrheal medications

Answer: c) Placing in contact isolation

Explanation: Placing a patient with Clostridium difficile infection in contact isolation helps prevent the spread of this highly contagious bacteria.

287. Q: What is a priority intervention for a patient with myasthenia gravis experiencing a crisis?

a) Administering anticholinesterase medications

b) Implementing fall precautions

c) Administering corticosteroids

d) Providing respiratory support

Answer: d) Providing respiratory support

Explanation: Patients with myasthenia gravis in crisis may experience respiratory muscle weakness. Providing respiratory support, such as ventilatory assistance, is crucial to maintain adequate breathing.

288. Q: Which dietary modification is most appropriate for a patient with gallstones?

 a) High-carbohydrate diet

 b) Low-fat diet

 c) High-protein diet

 d) Low-sodium diet

 Answer: b) Low-fat diet

Explanation: A low-fat diet is often recommended for patients with gallstones to reduce the risk of gallbladder contractions triggered by fatty foods.

289. Q: What is the primary nursing intervention for a patient experiencing a sickle cell crisis?

 a) Administering oxygen

 b) Administering pain medication

 c) Administering fluids

 d) Administering folic acid

 Answer: b) Administering pain medication

Explanation: Pain management is a primary intervention for a patient experiencing a sickle cell crisis due to severe pain associated with vaso-occlusive events.

290. Q: Which intervention is crucial for a patient with acute angle-closure glaucoma?

 a) Administering osmotic diuretics

 b) Administering anti-inflammatory medications

c) Administering beta-blockers

d) Performing eye exercises

Answer: a) Administering osmotic diuretics

Explanation: Administering osmotic diuretics, such as mannitol, is a priority in acute angle-closure glaucoma to reduce intraocular pressure quickly.

291. Q: What is the priority nursing intervention for a patient with compartment syndrome?

a) Elevating the affected limb

b) Applying a compression bandage

c) Administering anti-inflammatory medications

d) Preparing the patient for fasciotomy

Answer: d) Preparing the patient for fasciotomy

Explanation: Compartment syndrome is a surgical emergency. Preparing the patient for a fasciotomy is essential to relieve pressure within the affected compartment.

292. Q: Which nursing action is priority for a patient with a suspected bowel obstruction?

a) Administering laxatives

b) Administering antiemetic medications

c) Initiating nasogastric suction

d) Encouraging fluid intake

Answer: c) Initiating nasogastric suction

Explanation: Initiating nasogastric suction is a priority for a patient with a suspected bowel obstruction to decompress the gastrointestinal tract and reduce the risk of further complications.

293. Q: Which of the following is a priority for a patient with a chest tube that has been accidentally removed?

a) Reinserting the chest tube immediately

b) Covering the site with a sterile dressing

c) Applying a tight, occlusive dressing to the site

d) Administering pain medication

Answer: b) Covering the site with a sterile dressing

Explanation: Covering the site with a sterile dressing is essential to prevent air from entering the pleural space and to maintain proper chest tube function.

294. Q: What is the priority nursing intervention for a patient in malignant hyperthermia?

a) Administering dantrolene

b) Applying cooling blankets

c) Administering antipyretics

d) Monitoring vital signs every 15 minutes

Answer: a) Administering dantrolene

Explanation: Administering dantrolene is the priority in malignant hyperthermia to reverse the hypermetabolic state and prevent life-threatening complications.

295. Q: Which of the following is the most appropriate intervention for a patient with Parkinson's disease experiencing bradykinesia?

a) Administering levodopa/carbidopa

b) Administering anticholinergic medications

c) Implementing a regular exercise program

d) Administering muscle relaxants

Answer: a) Administering levodopa/carbidopa

Explanation: Administering levodopa/carbidopa is a primary intervention for managing bradykinesia in patients with Parkinson's disease.

296. Q: What is the priority nursing intervention for a patient experiencing a hemorrhagic stroke?

a) Administering anticoagulant medications

b) Maintaining a patent airway

c) Administering thrombolytic agents

d) Monitoring blood pressure levels

Answer: b) Maintaining a patent airway

Explanation: Maintaining a patent airway is a priority for a patient with a hemorrhagic stroke to ensure adequate oxygenation and ventilation.

297. Q: Which intervention is a priority for a patient with Bell's palsy?

a) Administering antiviral medications

b) Administering muscle relaxants

c) Providing eye protection

d) Implementing a soft diet

Answer: c) Providing eye protection

Explanation: Providing eye protection is crucial for patients with Bell's palsy, as they may have difficulty closing their eye completely, leading to eye dryness and injury.

298. Q: What is the most appropriate nursing action for a patient with a suspected upper GI bleed?

a) Initiating a proton pump inhibitor

b) Administering oral iron supplements

c) Performing guaiac test on stools

d) Administering vitamin K

Answer: a) Initiating a proton pump inhibitor

Explanation: Initiating a proton pump inhibitor is often part of the initial management for patients with upper gastrointestinal bleeding to reduce gastric acid production.

299. Q: What is the priority nursing action for a patient with Addison's disease experiencing a crisis?

a) Administering hydrocortisone

b) Monitoring blood glucose levels

c) Administering fludrocortisone

d) Encouraging a diet high in sodium

Answer: a) Administering hydrocortisone

Explanation: Administering hydrocortisone is essential during an Addison's disease crisis to replace deficient adrenal hormones.

300. Q: Which intervention is critical for a patient with an acute myocardial infarction?

a) Administering nitroglycerin

b) Administering beta-blockers

c) Administering morphine sulfate

d) Administering aspirin

Answer: d) Administering aspirin

Explanation: Administering aspirin is a critical intervention during an acute myocardial infarction to reduce platelet aggregation and minimize the size of the infarct.

Chapter Five

References

1. **NCLEX-PN Review Books:** The NCLEX-PN is the examination that LPNs (Licensed Practical Nurses) must pass to become licensed.

   - Saunders Comprehensive Review for the NCLEX-PN® Examination

   - Lippincott's Review for NCLEX-PN

2. **Nursing Textbooks:** Standard nursing textbooks can provide in-depth information on a variety of topics covered in the exam.

   - Fundamentals of Nursing by Patricia A. Potter and Anne Griffin Perry

   - Medical-Surgical Nursing: Assessment and Management of Clinical Problems by Sharon L. Lewis

3. **Pharmacology References:**

- Pharmacology: A Patient-Centered Nursing Process
  Approach by Linda E. McCuistion

4. **Anatomy and Physiology References:**

- Human Anatomy & Physiology by Elaine N. Marieb
  and Katja Hoehn

In the creation of this content, Artificial Intelligence (AI) was utilized as a tool to assist in generating material, providing insights, and offering suggestions. The AI's role was instrumental in developing the initial drafts of questions, answers, and explanatory content, which were subsequently meticulously reviewed, refined, and validated by me, the author, to ensure the accuracy and validity of each item. This process was crucial in maintaining the integrity and reliability of the content provided in this reviewer.

Following the creation of the initial content, I conducted a rigorous and extensive review, double-checking each question and answer against reputable references to guarantee their validity and correctness. This step is paramount in ensuring that each piece of information is correct and serves its educational purpose efficiently and effectively.

In addition to validating the content, I performed a meticulous plagiarism check using a sophisticated, paid plagiarism checker. This step was essential to affirm the originality and authenticity of the material, making certain it does not contain any unoriginal or plagiarized content. It is of utmost importance for users of this reviewer to be confident in the uniqueness and authenticity of the content they are studying.

It is important to note that, while AI was an invaluable resource in the content creation process, the final responsibility for the accuracy, quality, and validity of the content lies solely with me, the author.

Thus, this content should be considered as a collaborative effort between human creativity and expertise and artificial intelligence assistance, culminating in a product designed to aid learning and improve understanding.